Don't Lose Fat
~ Burn It!

If You Lose Something ~

*You Keep Looking Till
You Find It Again!*

If You Burn Something ~

*It's Dead and Gone
So You Move On!*

DISCLAIMER

Whenever considering weight loss or weight reduction programs, consult with your physician or healthcare provider. The information provided here is not intended to replace consultation or advice received from your doctor or qualified health professionals regarding your specific situation nor is it to be taken as medical advice or diagnosis. All information offered in this book are merely opinions regarding the diet proposed by Dr. Simeons. Losing 1 to 2 pounds a day is a result that many on the hCG diet have done, but is not a guarantee.

Luci *(aka)* Lucille Flint, and/or any of her affiliates, associates or independent contractors shall NOT assume any legal, monetary, or any other type of responsibility for your decision to use this book as a guideline in the use of hCG and the 500 calorie diet or for any other reasons.

Table of Contents

Dear Reader,

Please read this entire book before beginning any weight reduction (loss) program.

What you will learn could be the difference between failure and success.

You will learn information about the functions of your body you probably never knew, which could help you now . . . as well as in the future.

Sincerely with joy,

Luci (aka) *Lucille Flint*

Life is not what happens to you,

But how you react to it . . .

For what caused you to react

Will surely pass.

But how you continue to react

Can only be stopped by you.

~ Luci Flint

Introduction

Let's face it. Who wants to be fat? It's not only women, who don't want to be fat, but men, and teenagers too. Honestly, I don't believe anybody wants to be **fat**. Do you?

Think about the sub-title of this book for a moment and ponder the words.

Psychologically when 'something' is lost you subconsciously try to find it again. Let's say that 'something' is your fat. If you've had that 'something' (fat) for some time and you lose it, your whole system kicks in unconsciously without forethought and will attempt to find that 'something' (your fat).

After pondering this for some time I realized that this could be why the majority of people who 'lose' fat, gain it back again and again and again.

But if that 'something' (fat) is killed . . . by burning it up, your mind automatically knows that it is dead and gone and will not start searching for it. It knows

DEAD is DEAD and GONE is GONE. Your mind then let's it go, enabling you to get on with your life. Slim and shapely, be you a man, teen or woman.

It is a known fact that obesity has become epidemic virtually all over the world. Why?

I'm sure there are numerous reasons. One could be from watching too much TV. Have you noticed the media is continually bombarding you with ads about food and every sort of drug imaginable? The time has perhaps come to stop watching those food and drug ads on TV!

It's time to start controlling you and your diet. One that can and will change your body to the goal you set for yourself or need to set. You need a firm determination to get off the foods and/or drugs *(medications)* binge. Doing so could be a way for you to shape up and get healthy at the same time.

In order to accomplish that you need powerful strategies that will catapult you in the right direction.

One strategy you must realize is how important it is to get started on a sound nutritional program that will provide the results you are looking for. Just sitting in a chair and wishing for your body to get healthy and in shape won't cut it. You must make a decision; stick with it and **take action!**

Do not wait.

The time will

never

Be just right.

~ Napoleon Hill

Your time is not tomorrow

Your time is now!

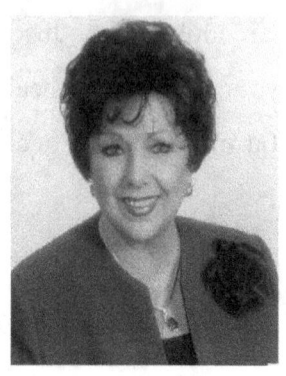

Luci's Creed

When I start on a path to achieve honest, sincere success . . . I will never, never, never give up, give in, nor quit! I will keep adjusting; climbing; helping others in their climb; learning; and succeeding one step at a time . . . I then will not only reach the top because of others I have helped who push me to the top, but because of my own efforts.

Luci (aka) Lucille Flint

DEDICATION

I dedicate this book to all who have struggled with being fat, obese, out of shape, and physically unwell due to the problems that haunt your every moment. I offer this book to you with love, concern, and sorrow for the years you have thus suffered.

My prayer is that you will find hope for your future with a newly found resolve to take control of your life.

And last but not least, my beloved husband, Don, our only child Jill, three granddaughters and their husbands and six beautiful great-grandchildren who affectionately call me GG.

Which twin read Luci's Book?

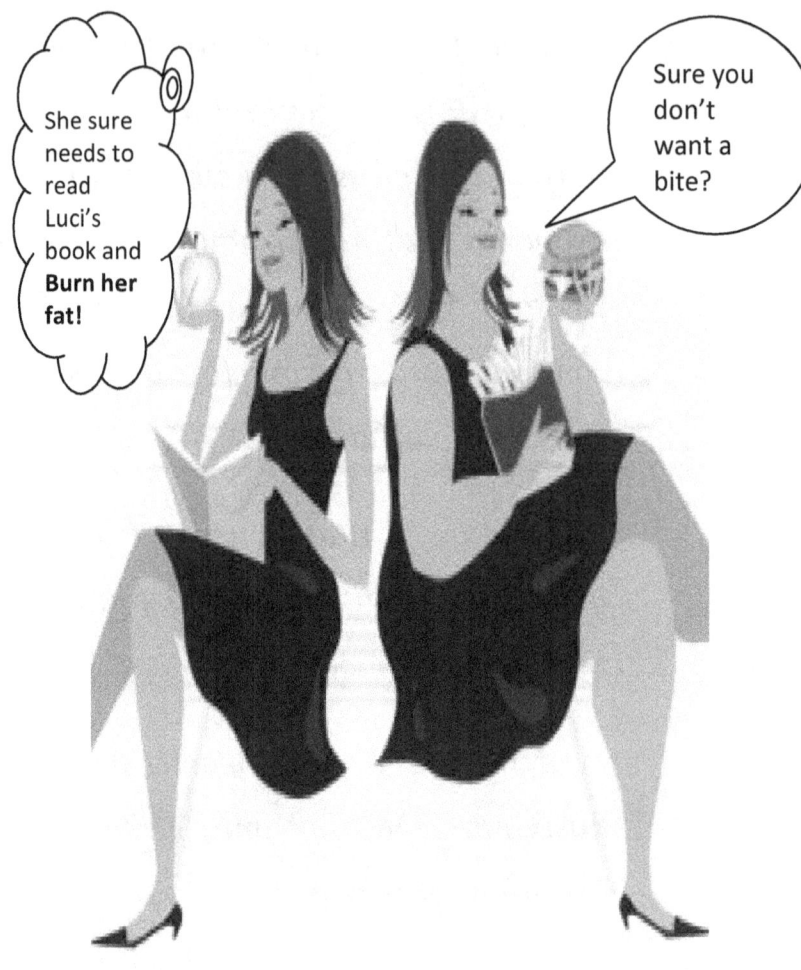

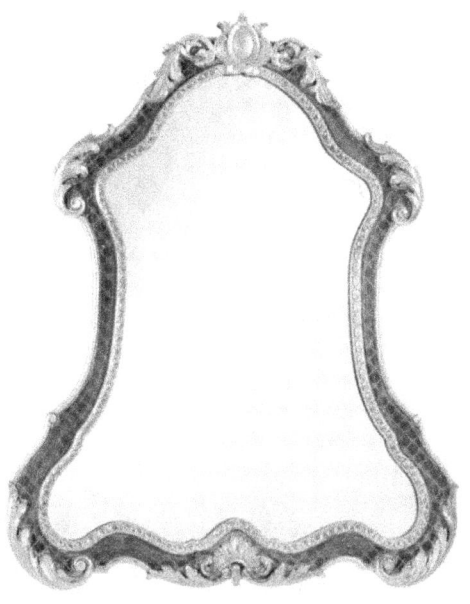

"LIFE IS JUST A MIRROR
AND WHAT YOU SEE OUT
THERE, YOU MUST FIRST
SEE INSIDE OF YOU"

~ Wally 'Famous' Amos

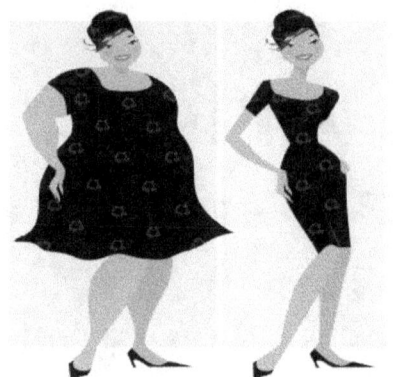 Women

Men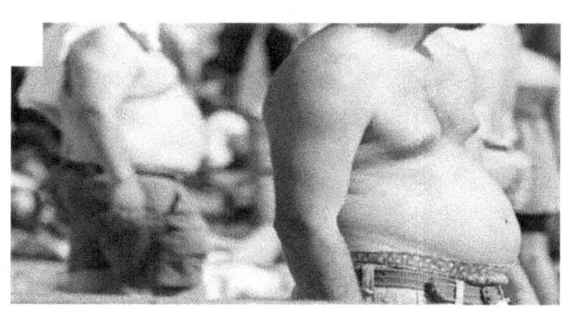

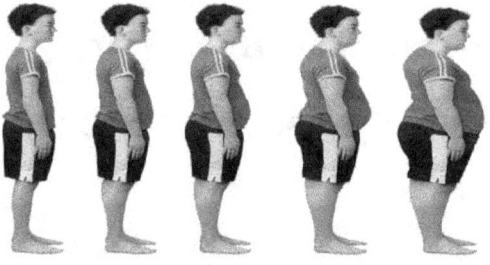 Teens

FIRST THINGS FIRST

Let me ask you a few questions?

1) How long have you been over weight?

2) How fast do you want to burn off your fat?

3) How serious are you about reducing your weight?

4) How do you expect to re-shape your body?

5) Is exercise in the picture?

6) What type of exercise can you physically do? What are your limitations, if any?

7) Find a picture of **yourself** *(not a model or someone else)* when you were at your ideal shape and weight. Scan it onto your computer and print it numerous times. Why? Because you need to tape it up on your bathroom mirror; on the door of the fridge; on the inside of your fridge; on the cabinet where you keep your special foods; in your car; in your day planner *(move it daily)*; on the table beside your chair where you watch TV; and any other place where you can continually see yourself as the person you **really are**! *(If you've never been slim, then take another*

picture of someone you admire and put your face on it).

8) You need to understand that to reduce your weight it normally includes a cost of some sort. Do you have enough money to get started and see it through to your ideal weight?

9) Before you make the decision whether you have the money or not, let me ask you to do a little simple project.

- Take a notebook and pen and for forty days, on a daily basis keep track of everything you eat and drink *(coffee, tea, sodas, liquor),* plus the amount of pure water.

- Put a cost beside each item on your list making sure you calculate all your drinks, snacks, purchased water, etc.

- When eating a meal with an assortment of foods served at the dinner table you will need to calculate the cost of the food and then divide it by how many servings resulted from the full amount. Weigh or measure the food you ate so you know the proportions, and can then calculate the cost.

- Add up the total cost daily and weekly. Then total the forty days. *(The forty days is the approximate length of this fat reduction plan. The amount $ will probably surprise you, it certainly did me).*

I believe you'll find **you do have the money** to obtain the necessary products and foods to accomplish your goals.

10) How long have you wanted to lose your fat?

11) Do you want to feel better physically and psychologically?

12) If you're a woman, do you want to feel desired, loved, appreciated and attractive?

13) If you're a man, do you also have those same feelings, plus you want to have back your powerful sex drive?

14) If you're a teenager, do you want to be accepted, liked, popular, and attractive?

It is really going to be up to you. I know you don't

want to be fat! If you have the desire and faith to take action, you can achieve your goal and quickly make your dreams come true.

By taking action and following the **rules** *(yes, there are always rules when change is desired).* You will see and feel the excitement as your excess fat starts melting off your body like cheese.

So pay attention and even highlight in this book what you are learning. You will be exposed to tips, strategies, and great ideas for right eating that will take you places you never thought were possible. You will learn a lot about the functions of your body and the effects those functions have on your desires, emotions, diseases, problems, and overall health.

Don't worry you won't have to eat low-carb, high protein, or even a lot of fat. Plus, you won't get any advice from wannebie professionals who have thrown their theories to you over the years.

Instead of doing something you will hate that drives you crazy why don't you do something you'll learn to love because you will see results very quickly?

At the same time it will help you to get healthy and put you back in shape. If you ever dreamed you could see yourself as an attractive, slim, shapely person compared to the person you presently are, you're in for a wonderful surprise. Just think, if you follow the protocol that you'll learn about later in the book, in a short 45 days *(6 ½ weeks – 1 ½ months)* you could be a whole new you.

I will reveal how I got back in great shape and how I believe you can too. **See yourself** looking, feeling, and performing at your ultimate best, that of the slim, shapely person you will be.

The first step is to make a firm unchangeable commitment that you will stick to the protocol as outlined. Next you must **take responsibility** for your eating and fitness program.

I can promise you that life will be much happier, calmer, and more rewarding when you take care of yourself correctly.

Let me tell you the secret
that has led me to my goal
My strength lies solely in
my tenacity.

~ Louis Pasteur

Yesterday I dared

to struggle.

Today I dare to win~

~ Bernadette Devlin

What Is At Stake - Your Life?

"If you don't take care of yourself,

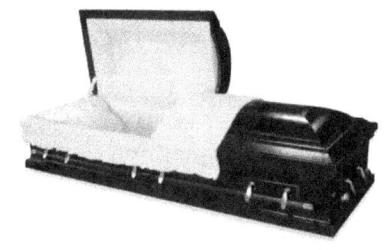

The undertaker will take over

That responsibility for you. "

~ Carrie Latet

Before I begin with the 'program or protocol' I want to digress a bit and explain the seriousness of getting your health in order. The health condition of the majority of people in developed nations has deteriorated to such an extent that it has literally become a serious worldwide crisis. It is a **'Fat Epidemic'**.

Research shows that 75% of people in America are obese because they mostly eat fatty food such as takeaways! Add 15% for people who are considered only fat not obese. By adding the two statistics together, the fat epidemic adds up to 90%. *(I'm not sure how the researchers come up with those statistics . . . which to me sounds exceptionally high. I only know that I **was** one of those in the statistic).* This is a sad fact and something that needs to change.

Do you think that the normal way to live is to be out of shape, overweight, and have all kinds of diseases? **It truly is insanity!**

To think that nine out of ten *(that is 90%)* people are either fat or obese is a terrible stat. This is also what is happening all over the world in developed nations. I've thought a lot about all this and have come to the basic conclusion that through the last fifty plus years we have followed the so-called experts who promoted many different theories or postulations about what we should or should not eat for our health and wellbeing.

I think of the lowly 'egg' and how we've been told for years to avoid them like the plague due to the high amount of cholesterol in them. We **now know** that the cholesterol in the egg **does not cause** a buildup of cholesterol in your arteries, but actually helps reduce cholesterol attributed mostly to the naturally occurring lecithin in the egg. You should never fry them in butter, margarine, or other fats or oils. Of course when you eat breakfast out, the restaurants normally use one of those fats for cooking eggs, unless you specify differently.

You should eat them only if they are soft or hard boiled. If you must fry them, then use an organic, cold-pressed virgin coconut oil with its medium chain triglycerides *(MCT)* which does not add to your fat.

Almost on a daily basis science is now proving that many of the eating guidelines of the past such as with the egg and a plethora of other foods was totally wrong and actually has contributed to the many ailments and diseases as a result of being obese or just fat.

What this comes down to, is that it is up to you to make your own change in your food choices. It can be done! But it can only be done 'one person at a time'. You are the one responsible for your life and how you choose to live it. No matter how you would like to push the blame on someone else *(mom, dad, genetics, etc)*, the fact is that '**no one else is to blame or responsible**'. You are the decision maker.

You must understand right now that no one is going to help you, except yourself. You are the master of your decisions, thoughts, actions and re- actions. You have to stop eating junk food; drinking damaging dangerous pep-up drinks and sodas; or popping pills of every sort. You must begin consuming nutritious foods and drinking lots of water.

The trillion dollar food manufacturing business won't help you. The billion dollar health industry won't help you. Even mega-trillion dollar drug companies and medical establishment won't help you. Why should they? It could only mean a loss of revenue for them. After all the world runs on **money!**

Have you ever thought or wondered why there are so many commercials on TV sponsoring fast foods? The simple fact is they are offering you inexpensive foods with the convenience of a drive-thru for people with busy schedules, which fattens their wallets and your middle. It's a catch-22 scenario with its vicious cycle of poor eating habits, then using a supposedly 'quick fix' weight loss drink or a bunch of pills.

Another reason so many are getting fat and obese is because most live a sedentary lifestyle. Few walk anymore. Instead we drive everywhere. Kids are not spending their time running around and playing games outside. Instead, they sit down with their video games; or spend time surfing the internet; or on their telephone chatting or texting with their friends. Yes, I know adults are guilty of this too.

(To help you know if you're obese or just fat . . . you can check the standard Body Mass Index (BMI) Chart in the Bibliography section at the end of the book).

Eating and Drinking

It seems many people are getting fatter or becoming obese not only because of the foods they eat but also how fast they consume their meals. Much of your food is never digested nor is the nutrition assimilated and utilized by your body because it is not chewed properly or long enough. For best results you should chew your food at least twenty-five times before swallowing it. Also far too many people gulp down their food by drinking *(usually a soda)* during their meals. This should be restricted as much as possible. Drink before eating or about an hour after your meal.

Another problem is that far too many items bought from the stores are processed and refined. Most foods are loaded with chemicals to preserve them for shelf life. You live in a fast-paced world. You grab quick junk food from corner stores, fast food joints, and restaurants. Why? Because you claim you don't have time to cook or you're too tired to plan and cook a nutritious meal for yourself or your family. No wonder you're tired, look what you eat and how it's cooked.

While talking about cooked or cooking foods, let me reveal some information I learned years ago.

Microwave Ovens

Yes, I know we all love them because they are so convenient, easy, and fast. However, let me reveal some information you probably don't know, nor will you see it ever publicized again.

Years ago before microwave ovens became available to the public they had to be tested. Home economists working with the scientists took a great variety of foods to cook in the microwave ovens. They were to test the foods for taste, texture, and timing. The microbiologists were to determine these same finding and also check if the nutritional value was still intact. The microbiologists found that indeed the 'microwaved' foods did retain a good texture and taste. And yes, the vitamins, some minerals and amino acids *(all enzymes were gone)* were still intact as far as their molecular structure was concerned. But the energy in the actual nutrients had **become inert** *(in other words lifeless)* after being cooked in the microwave. This information was quickly squashed due to the powerful lobbyist and money changing hands. It could have been disastrous to the industry on both sides of the coin.

I wonder if they ever gave you and me, along with the rest of the consumers a thought as to our nutritional needs. In other words the nutrition appeared to still be in tact under the microscope of those microwaved foods, but the activity which gives us the **live nutrition with energy was dead** *(inert)*.

Most of the public is totally unaware of these facts as we use our microwave ovens more and more. Restaurants even micro much of the food they serve.

Sure the food tastes basically the same as it fills you up, but the **nutritional energy from the food is lacking**. Is it any wonder that most people complain of lack of energy and are always tired? Too many children are either lack luster or are overly active being diagnosed with ADD/ADHD. The vicious cycle goes on and on and on.

The plain and simple fact is that too many of us have become lazy, lackadaisical or maybe don't realize the consequences of how critical it is to plan, shop, properly cook, and serve a nutritious meal to yourself and your family on a day-to-day basis. Your total health and wellbeing are dependent on it.

In order to get out of that rut you need to understand that **you are in control**. You can and must act responsibly. *(You'll find more research on micros in my FREE OFFER, see page 143).*

Irradiation

Many of our foods are being irradiated so they stay fresh longer. Do you know what they are irradiated with? Most likely you don't, but I'll tell you. They are irradiated with atomic fusion waste. That's right; the powers that be decided they didn't know what to do with the waste *(or where to store it since it is extremely dangerous, unstable and deadly).* Those scientists knew that radiation killed bacteria and virtually everything else that is bombarded with it. So they made the decision that it was just what the producers and processors of our food supply needed.

For instance they could radiate potatoes so they would last longer in shipment and stay on the store shelves in fresh like condition. **That process is called irradiation.** *(Potatoes are just one of the many items irradiated).*

Years ago, I was part a group from the NNFA who endeavored to get the FDA to enact a law demanding the producers label the foods that had been irradiated. But as far as I know the law was never enacted. I don't recall ever seeing a sign up in the grocery stores that states a product has been 'irradiated'. Have you?

Did they consider what it would do to you and me? Of course not! Perhaps all they saw or considered were dollar signs in their eyes if they sold the **atomic fusion waste** to the food producers and processors; who then saw more dollar signs in their eyes by keeping their produce or foods from spoiling as rapidly. Again, did they care about you and me? I think not!

Get back to basics!

Some of you might ask, 'what basics'? Especially you younger generations who are currently raising your families. What are those basics that many of you may have never learned?

If you fit into this category you need to study and learn how to plan nutritious meals, and then shop for the best buys of quality fresh fruits, produce, meats, and grains. Learn to cook them properly and serve them to your family. It's great when a young couple can work on this project together.

If you have no one to teach you, look on the internet. You could attend classes taught in relationship to foods, cooking and nutrition by many health food stores or specialty shops that sponsor **free workshops**.

Changing Habits Can Help Prevent Weight Gain.

Most of you might **not believe** that changing your habits for shopping, cooking, and serving delicious meals to your family could help with the solution of being overweight **or** that it just couldn't be that simple. Who knows, you might be right, but it would help break a pattern of unhealthy eating, which could help tremendously with weight control while enhancing you and your family's health, happiness and relationships. When you and your family are healthy and happy you don't have to be continually stressed or worried about your health. Or with the added burden of grief and sorrow from excessive diseases, illnesses, and many times death. Think also of the cost . . . which can tear a person apart mentally, physically and monetarily.

Burning Fat

I know the current issue is to **burn fat.** However, first I feel you need is to have more facts about the functioning of your body before you undertake your fat reduction plan. Then you need to **take action**. I have found that when a person understands the reasoning behind their action they have a tendency to stay on track. A change needs to take place in your habits, thinking and metabolism so your **fat can melt off** while your inches are decreasing almost immediately.

You need to know **'the plan'** for your food choices; shopping and preparing your meals; and the importance of gentle exercise. Our bodies were meant to move about. This means physical work or moderate exercise. If you learn these facts and understand more about you bodily functions, you should not have to worry about being fat in the future.

If you are ready to learn how to get yourself in shape to develop a healthy body, prepare for an exciting journey. You are going to get an education for a lifetime. In the next chapter I'll reveal how I **burned up my fat~**

My Story

I GOT TIRED OF BEING F-A-T!

In order for you to get where you wanted to be, I am going to introduce to you the way I lost over 42 pounds *(3 stone or 19 kilos)* **in just 40+ days.** I had found a new way of eating that helped me **burn** the unhealthy and unwanted fat, inches, and pounds that I had built-up over the last 15 or so years.

I'll never forget after I started to gain a good bit of weight that my darling husband said to me in a very loving and kind way ~ "Sweetheart, you're much too pretty to be fat".

Did those words hurt? Of course they did, but the way he said them, I knew he was only trying to encourage me to lose the weight in his kind and loving way. And that is exactly what I tried to do, over and over again.

Oh yes, I had tried all types of weight loss modalities during those years. Special diets, pills, drinks, juices, exercise, exercise equipment, patches, will power and mind control. You bet I tried them all!

Did they all work? The truth is that yes, to a point. I did lose some weight. ***Remember when you lose something, your whole system kicks into find it again and again.*** Even with extremely dedicated effort, I did lose some weight, but I **never** got my shape back. I tried to get my shape back way before I started this protocol and nothing worked. I still wanted it back regardless of my age of 75 *(2010)*.

I wanted to wear my beautiful clothes again, wear my high heels *(I'll admit I'm a shoe freak, and yes, a classic clothes freak too)*. I wanted to feel good about myself knowing that not only did I look good but I felt great too.

I wanted my belly fat gone! I wanted to **burn off** the fat. I wanted those excess inches off my hips, thighs and upper arms to disappear.

After years of frustration, disappointment, regret, anger at myself, and a plethora of emotions I finally knew I had to try a completely different course of action . . . just **one more time** I told myself. So here's what I did.

After seeing others who seemed to suddenly and almost magically slim down and reshape, I knew I had to find out how and what they had done or were doing.

My journey began by talking to friends I trusted who had regained their shape by burning off their excessive fat. I asked a lot questions and from what I heard, I knew I needed to do a lot of research.

Because of my interest in nutrition and microbiology, which began back in the late 1950's I've always been prone to research. I am a dedicated, self-educated researcher in nutrition, microbiology, and virtually every type of health modality. I have enjoyed and learned from vast resources that became available to me. I have been introduced to and taken advantage of their training and learning throughout my life. I still am an avid advocate for healthy living, which includes nutritious well cooked and attractively served meals.

So why and how did I gain so much weight?

You will be able to read more about how I began to gain weight in my soon to be published book

Nine Lives

Volumes 1, 2 and 3

A tale of excitement, sorrow, adventure, deceit and greed while treading into unknown territories in a fascinating journey to joy and peace.

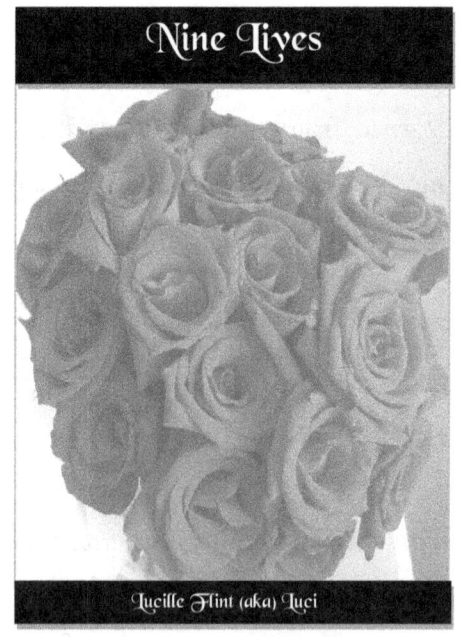

A New Course of Action and a Totally Radical Change of Thought

You'll learn a little later in the story what I heard and then how I researched all I could before making my final decision. After that I was willing to give it a go, so to speak.

It truly was a radical change for me to try a well known product, one that was considered a **fad** and controversial by the drug and medical establishments, as well as other companies who are in the diet industry. That didn't really concern me, as I understood their basic reasoning.

There were a few doctors who fully approved of the product and who would write a prescription for you. That is, after you answered a plethora of questions; gave you a brief exam *(some do it over the phone)*; attend an orientation and instruction class *(again sometimes over the phone)*; and signing a waiver not to hold the physician or his staff responsible.

I wasn't exactly sure as to why those doctors decided to jump into the field; yet I realized they knew there would be a tremendous need to help overweight people. And I'm not so naïve as to believe that those doctors who jumped on the band wagon realized there would be a lot of money earned for their services.

I also wondered if they had really studied about the product. I don't know, but it didn't really matter to me, because after my research, analyzing and study I figured I would try the program.

I'll tell you this was a serious and major decision for me to make. A decision I would have shunned and strongly advised against years previously. After feeling assured about the protocol I made an appointment with the recommended physician *(MD)*, which was within a short driving distance from my home.

It's not hard to make decisions
When you know what your
values are.

~ *Roy Disney*

Intriguing - What I Found Out

Perhaps you have heard of hCG by now as it seems to be a hot commodity and subject. It's all over Facebook, Twitter, YouTube and Social Groups. I can certainly understand why, because it really works if you follow the diet protocol exactly and use the true hCG injectable product as used by Dr. Simeons, who discovered, researched and used hCG for weight reduction with a diet protocol.

What Is hCG? Your Understanding is Important!

hCG stands for 'Human Chorionic Gonadotropin', and is a glycoprotein or hormone composed of 244 amino acids. Not to be confused with hGH *(Human Growth Hormone).*

Dr. Simeons found hCG to be the **'Key'** that unlocks the body's **'Abnormal Fat'** reserves as an energy source. It is the abnormal fat that you want to **burn.**

hCG is created primarily during the first trimester of pregnancy by every woman or female animal. It is actually the hormone that is responsible for affecting whether or not you get a negative or plus sign in a home pregnancy test. During pregnancy, hCG assists the mother in preparation for the development of the baby. Without hCG, the mother would not be able to provide the energy that a growing baby demands. hCG assists the mother by metabolizing fats at a rapid enough pace so all the energy demands for the development of the baby will be met. It may not seem like a lot at first glance, but building an entire baby in 9 months is a big job. This is why hCG is so effective. Not only does hCG help to metabolize energy stores, but it also prepares the mother by assisting in the balancing of her current hormone imbalances while pregnant.

Dr. A. T.W. Simeons, M.D.,
the genius behind hCG.

Over fifty years ago, Dr. Simeons pioneered a revolutionary new approach to weight reduction.

The controversial usage of hCG is as an adjunct to the British endocrinologist Dr. A.T.W. Simeons, M.D. program coupled with an ultra-low-calorie weight-reduction diet of 500 calories during the protocol period. Unlike many other weight loss programs the hCG protocol is not just a regular diet and exercise program, but rather a prescribed hCG protocol for medical intervention in weight reduction.

What Is To Blame?

Most programs incorporate a negative calorie deficit and exercise in an attempt to force the body into burning enough calories to lose weight. A problem with this is that there are usually more factors associated with why the individual who is overweight to begin with. It is believed by most that obesity is a condition brought about by unhealthy living. This may be true the majority of the time, yet there could be a heredity factor or both.

Have you ever stopped to figure out what the 'heredity factor is'? Generally speaking, it is one generation acting, cooking and eating what the previous generations had done that caused them to be fat. Generational habits are all virtually the same and are hard to break. That is why hCG works so well because it helps to re-set or changes your metabolism regardless of your generational behavior. This is done by the change that takes place with your metabolism initiated by the hCG.

The hCG diet predominantly **burns fat** as compared to lean body mass, which is where other weight loss programs fail. Not only does the hCG protocol burn a higher percentage of fat as compared to other diets, but it also accomplishes it in a fraction of the time. hCG people burn an average of 3/4 to 1 pound a day and can expect to reduce as much weight in **one day** that most other diets and weight loss programs accomplish in **one week**. Also, the weight reduction during the hCG program is kept off better as the body's natural set-point is re-established.

How Dr. Simeons Discovered Fat Burning

While studying pregnant women in India on a calorie deficient diet and 'fat boys' with pituitary problems, Dr. Simeons discovered when he treated the 'fat boys' with low-doses of hCG, he discovered it burned fat rather than lean *(muscle)* tissue. He reasoned that hCG must be re-programming the **hypothalamus**. Much like with the pregnant mother the naturally occurring hCG protects the developing fetus by promoting mobilization and consumption of abnormal, excessive adipose deposits *(abnormal fat.)*

Dr. Simeons realized that hCG was resetting the hypothalamus *(more about how it functions a little later).* His patients were burning abnormal fat and they seemed healthier and happier. Gone were the extremes in personality and moods. **Something good was really happening.**

Dr. Simeons, while practicing at Salvator Mundi International Hospital in Rome, Italy recommended a daily low-dose hCG injection in combination with a customized ultra-low-calorie *(500 calories a day, high-protein, low-carbohydrate/fat)* diet for reduction of adipose tissue without the loss of lean tissue. **The results were astounding.**

After Dr. Simeons' death, the diet started to spread to specialized centers via popularization by such individuals as the author Kevin Trudeau, a specialist in promotion.

Choices are the hinges of destiny

The foods you eat today . . .

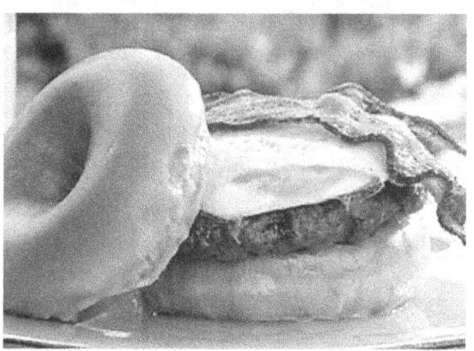

Will be what you feel and see tomorrow.

What you see and feel tomorrow will be
who and what you become in your future.

What you are in your future

Will be how and if you will enjoy a

Life full of wellness and freedom or

A life of dis-ease the rest of you days.

~ Luci Flint

Controversy and My Belief

After hCG became rapidly popular because of the great success in burning fat and weight reduction a controversy soon developed. In an article the Journal of the American Medical Association *(JAMA)* and the American Journal of Clinical Nutrition *(AJCN)* began issuing warnings against the use of hCG, saying that the hCG was neither safe, nor effective as a weight-loss aid.

I feel I must comment on that paragraph. For myself, I believe only a very small portion of what any article would say or reveal that is printed in the JAMA or the AJCN. It seems there have been far too many fraudulent articles written for a payoff by highly accredited researchers and physicians. More and more of those types of revelations are coming out and being reported. In fact there have been several revealed by the press in 2009.

I know from past experience that many of those magazine articles and statements are from various contributors, who are really offering only their opinions instead of a scientific set of facts. Most have never done actual studies or tests regarding the product which they have written or spoken about. It was after those articles came out that the majority of doctors, nutritionist and others jumped on the **'do not use hCG'** band wagon. They never bothered to research or study the facts. Like sheep they followed others blindly into the abbess.

I have been involved and around medical communities for decades. I feel I understand why the above mentioned organizations would come out against hCG. Could the following be a few reasons as to why they are normally so against the studies and tests such as those completed by Dr. Simeons?

- They or one of their colleagues didn't discover the use of hCG.

- Perhaps they don't see how they could make any money from those studies.

- The studies came from a foreign country, which in decades past it seemed that the 'powers that be' didn't readily accept such studies. Too many have been and still are a group of elitists.

True, they probably are among the best in the world, but many other doctors and research scientists from other countries have added greatly to their knowledge.

- Perhaps the drug companies didn't see how they could reproduce hCG chemically, patent it and still retain the same results for burning fat.

- Who knows what else goes through their minds. I question as to whether those nay-sayers' ever studied hCG or the hypothalamus? I wonder if they have done physical and practical research on the use of hCG for fat and weight reduction. I doubt it, because if they did, they might have to admit that Dr. Simeons was right.

What Others Are Saying

Many individuals believe that the results found through the use of hCG are too good to be true. Often hCG providers take little caution when making claims about the positive effects of hCG.

Although there have been enormous claims about the use of hCG for healing just about every illness imaginable, it could be mostly in the imagination. Yet when a person gets healthier all sorts of good things can happen. It did seem that some of the stories were a little farfetched.

With what scientific background I've had it was hard for me to believe some of those stories I heard. But after reviewing the evidence and researching the actions and re-actions of the hypothalamus plus understanding the physiology of the body I knew that it was possible that some of the stories could be true.

I learned that the hypothalamus could be re-programmed, and your metabolism changed so it would **burn fat**. I was convinced that a person could reduce their weight; the fat would come off; the inches reduced; re-shaping would take place, which would account for a much healthier person.

I realized that Dr Simeons had truly **pioneered a revolutionary** new approach to weight reduction that is much more powerful for **burning fat** at a rapid rate than any other weight loss plan ever developed and on the market today.

Common sense in an uncommon degree

Is what the world calls Wisdom.

~ Samuel Taylor Coleridge

It's my belief that Dr. Simeons had that wisdom.

So I picked a field where I had a little exposure.

Where I could have an enormous challenge

And have a chance to really do some good.

To be a pioneer in an area

And not just be like everyone else.

~ Henry Kravis

I believe that Dr. Simeons may have done just that without consciously realizing it at the time.

The important thing is not to stop questioning.

Curiosity has its own reason for existing.

One cannot help but be in awe when he contemplates the mysteries of eternity, of life, of the marvelous structure of reality.

It is enough if one tries merely to comprehend a little of this mystery every day.

Never lose a holy curiosity

~ Albert Einstein

Hypothalamus in Control

(hī-pó-thăl-ă-mŭs)

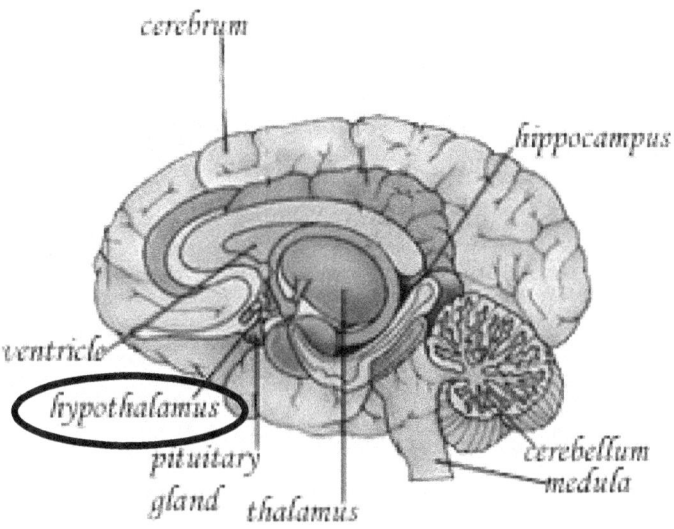

Here you can see where the hypothalamus is located and realize how small it is it. When you learn how powerful and dependent your body is on this tiny gland you should be extremely impressed.

Now let me reveal to you why the hypothalamus is **so critical.** You'll learn what happens when it **functions properly**, and what happens when **it doesn't**.

I know I'm giving you a rather lengthy explanation about the function and importance of your hypothalamus. I also realize that some of you might skip over the information, **please don't**. I truly believe it is critically important for you to understand the function of your hypothalamus. Hopefully this information will help you understand what is going on within your body. If you have a better understanding you might not get into a panic and believe the direst scenarios when problems start taking place with your body or system. Panic and fear can cause a wide swing in your emotions, which will cause even more dysfunction of all your glands and hormones.

After many years of research and practice I honestly believe that if people had a better understanding about the functions of their body they wouldn't panic; and begin taking all sorts of prescriptions, elixirs, herbs, juices, drugs or medicines that could do more harm than good. As I listen to the drugs possible side effects I wonder sometimes why anyone would take them. It seems like some of the side effects are worse than the original problem. Of course, that's just my opinion, as everyone has to make their own decision.

No Guessing Game

If you have doubts about what is going on with your body don't play the guessing game. By all means go to your physician and have yourself tested for those specific concerns.

Unless there is something **seriously wrong** you might give more thought about taking a lot of prescription drugs 'just in case'. Too many times it seems that the 'just in case' never happens, especially if the situation is given a little time to cure itself. Again be aware of the plethora of serious and dangerous side-effects of any drug.

What Is The Hypothalamus?

The hypothalamus is the control center of all autonomic regulatory activities of the body. **It has been said that the hypothalamus is the brain of the brain.** It is the hub for automatic and endocrine homeostatic systems such as cardiovascular, temperature, and abdominal visceral regulation. It manages all endocrine hormonal levels, sensory processing, and organizing the body metabolism, as well as ingestive behaviors. It appears that almost everything the hypothalamus does is related in some way to the management of brain and body connection, linking the psyche *(mind)* to the body.

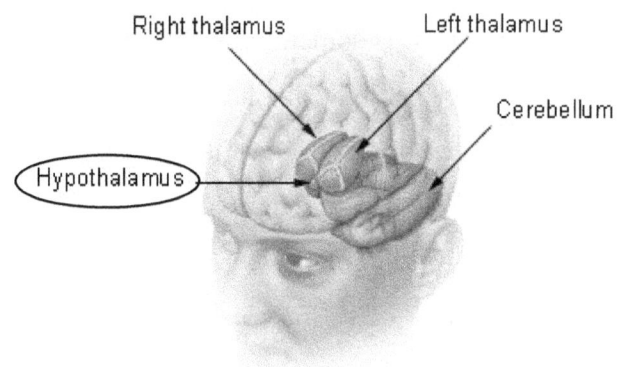

What Does The Hypothalamus Really Do?

The **hypothalamus** is a portion of the **brain** that contains a number of small **nuclei** with a variety of functions. One of the most important functions of the hypothalamus is to link the **nervous system** to the **endocrine system** via the **pituitary gland** *(hypothesis)*.

You can see the location of the hypothalamus which is

located below the **thalamus,** just above the **brain stem. It is roughly the size of an almond.** The hypothalamus is responsible for certain **metabolic** processes and other activities of the **Autonomic Nervous System.** It synthesizes and secretes **neurohormones,** often called hypothalamic-releasing hormones, and these in turn stimulate or inhibit the secretion of **pituitary hormones.** The hypothalamus controls **body temperature, hunger, thirst, fatigue,** and **circadian** *(sleep)* **cycles.**

Very simply, the hypothalamus organizes and controls many complex **emotions, feelings and moods,** as well as all motivational states including **hunger, appetite and food intake, and everything to do with the concept of pleasure including satisfaction, comfort and creative activities.** The neurons in the hypothalamus produce a number of hypothalamic neurotransmitters which relay information and instruction to all parts of the brain and body directly influencing the pituitary gland, the growth hormone; thyroid hormone releasing factor; and other neuropeptides that are released via hypothalamic input.

The hypothalamus *(within the Cerebral Hemispheres)* is intimately involved in the integration of all physiological stimulation of all **five senses,** including

taste, smell, sight, sound, and **touch**. Which then translates, distills and assembles a moment in time into one discernible 'package' relating all the attributes of an experience and all the associated stimulation into one clear harmonious concept, one memory, one experience. Thus it yields a succinct emotionally satisfying understanding and judgment of the experience.

The Hypothalamus Functions

The hypothalamus co-ordinates many hormonal and behavioral circadian rhythms, complex patterns of neuroendocrine outputs, complex homeostatic mechanisms, and many important behaviours.

The hypothalamus must therefore respond to many different signals, some of which are generated externally and some internally. It is thus richly connected with many parts of the **central nervous system**, including the brainstem **reticular formation** and **autonomic** zones, the limbic forebrain *(particularly the amygdala)*.

In general functions *(not all are listed)* of the

hypothalamus are of extreme importance for the functioning of your body, emotions, memory, general activity, and overall wellbeing. Such as:

1) Anxiety

2) Bladder *(contraction)*

3) Blood bone stimuli

4) Blood pressure *(decrease)*

5) Body temperature *(upward)*

6) Control for ADD/ADHD

7) Depression

8) Digestion

9) Eating reflexes

10) Energy levels

11) Gastric reflexes

12) Glucose regularity

13) Heart rate *(decrease)*

14) Hormonal/Neurotransmitter regulation

15) Hunger and Thirst

16) Hydration

17) Immune responses

18) Maternal behavior

19) Memory

20) Metabolism

21) Mood and Behavioral functions

22) Ovarian function

23) Pituitary gland regulation

24) PMS

25) Sleep *(circadian)* cycles

26) Smell *(olfactory stimuli)* including pheromones

27) Steroids *(gondola steroids and corticosteroids)*

28) Stress related disorders

29) Testicular function

30) Wakefulness

31) Water preservation

The hypothalamus is not considered an endocrine system but a neuroendocrine system.

Science has long recognized that in order for the brain to function properly and for the neurotransmitters in the brain to receive messages, the hypothalamus must be working properly. It is the functioning center for four of the brains most powerful hormones *(neurotransmitters)* that affect the mind.

Those powerful hormones are:

Serotonin – *among things it is thought to be involved in neural mechanisms important in sleep and sensory perception.*

Dopamine – *is used experimentally in treating hypotension and shock.*

Norepinephrine – *is chiefly a vaso-constrictor but has little effect on the cardiac output.*

Acetylcholine – *is thought to play an important role in the transmission of nerve impulses at synapses and myoneural junctions. Either excessive or deficient action of acetylcholine at the motor end-plates may result in a neuromuscular block.*

Most scientist and researchers believe that the improperly hypothalamic function could be the cause of most of the mental problems/chemical imbalances that affect children and adults.

The main function of the hypothalamus is to maintain the body's status quo. Factors such as blood pressure, body temperature, electrolyte and fluid balance, and **body weight** are held to a precise value called the set-point. Although this set-point can migrate over time, from day to day it is remarkably fixed.

Perhaps we all need to renew and empower the vital functions of our mind.

"The Cocoon drops off . . . The Caterpillar dies so
The Butterfly can be born.
Transform yourself from the unshapely
Cocoon and Caterpillar encased in a fat body.
Escape and shed it now! Left up your spirit as the

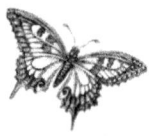

Wings of a Butterfly and soar to your
'Happy Ending'

~ Luci Flint

Hypothalamus Out of Control

What Happens When It Doesn't Work Properly?

Your hypothalamus is small yet it is perhaps the **most important part of your brain**. Your hypothalamus is your body's 'biological clock' - your 'circadian rhythm' that changes your mental and physical characteristics according to whether it's night or day. What's interesting is that **your hypothalamus needs natural daylight** in order to work properly.

If you're housebound or bedridden with perhaps Chronic Fatigue Syndrome, then the likelihood is that you probably don't get much natural daylight at all. In fact, **if you don't get more than two natural daylight hours - outdoors – every day** then you're likely to be suffering from **Natural Light Deficiency** *(NLD)*.

Research suggests that Chronic Fatigue Syndrome and Fibromyalgia sufferers have a disturbance in their hypothalamus . . . but in addition to that, they don't even get enough of the daylight needed to keep their hypothalamus working properly anyway. Is it really any wonder why your body clock and sleep might be all messed up if you have Chronic Fatigue Syndrome or Fibromyalgia?

When the hypothalamus is not working correctly, or up to par, so to speak, it generates and sends out the wrong neuro-signals, which are generated and then wrong neuro-messages are received. This reaction results in an inaccurate integration of all your sensory input leading to faulty perceptions which are very subtle but nonetheless powerful making you feel physically empty, deprived, emotionally and physically 'unsatisfied'. Dysfunction of the hypothalamus often leads to depression, obesity, hyperactivity, abnormal responses to stress, or disturbances in brain and limbic functioning.

Some physical aspects of hypothalamic dysfunction are:

1) Altered body temperatures

2) Autonomic dysfunction

3) Blood flow and blood pressure out of sync

4) Body out of harmony

5) Disordered sleep

6) Emotional imbalance

7) Energy imbalance

8) Immune dysfunction

9) Multiple hormonal dysfunctions *(Could this have something to do with lack of sex drive or libido?)*

10) Obsessive eating and weight gain

11) Temperature out of control *(too hot or cold)*

12) And many other functions, too numerous to list.

What causes dysfunction in the hypothalamus?

There can be numerous causes for dysfunction and symptoms which are:

1) Anorexia

2) Bleeding

3) Body temperature problems

4) Bulimia

5) Cold intolerance

6) Constipation

7) Depressed mood

8) Dizziness

9) Emotional problems

10) Excess thirst

11) Fatigue

12) Genetic disorders

13) Growths *(tumors)*

14) Hair or skin changes

15) Head trauma

16) Hoarseness

17) Impotence

18) Inability to smell

19) Infections and swelling *(inflammation)*

20) Loss of body hair and muscle *(in men)*

21) Lowered function of sexual hormones

22) Malnutrition

23) Mental slowing

24) Menstrual cycle changes

25) Obesity/Fat

26) Radiation

27) Surgery

28) Too much iron in the blood

29) Uncontrolled urination

30) Weakness

31) Weight gain

It's all a vicious cycle as to results of the functions or non-functions. The function of these vital systems can be altered by various causes ranging from food mishandling *(overeating);* dependency and substance *(drugs)* abuse and withdrawal; stress or psychological responses to simple functional deficits; hyperactivity; hypoactivity; environmental; or learning disabilities.

Unfortunately, hypothalamic function becomes impaired with age. So as you grow older the hypothalamus needs support to maintain optimum performance. With the understanding from all the previous lists, you might know that a hypothalamus dysfunction could attribute to the weight gain especially as you get older or 'Senior Moments'?

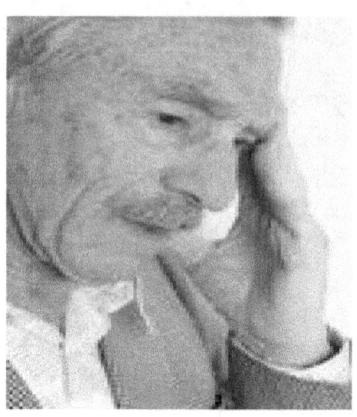

Maybe not remembering is not so bad . . . perhaps we forget all those unpleasant memories and are just happy to be alive!

If you want to test your memory, try to recall what you were worrying about one year ago today.

Without accepting the fact that everything changes, we cannot find perfect composure. But unfortunately, although it is true, it is difficult to accept it.
Because we cannot accept the truth of transience, we suffer.   ~Shunryu Suzuk

Different Types of Human Fat

There are three types of fat in the body: **Structural Fat**, **Normal Fat**, and **Abnormal Fat**. The fat we are most concerned about is the Abnormal Fat. This is the stuff that gets on our bodies and it just doesn't want to come off no matter how hard we try!

Structural Fat

Structural fat is vital for the smooth operation of the body. It is that fat that surrounds and protects your internal organs and provides the cushion on your feet so you can walk without pain. We need this kind of fat.

Normal Fat Reserves

This is the kind of fat that is just under your skin. It is called subcutaneous fat. The body can freely use it and store it without any problem. Most adults can have about 10 - 20 pounds of normal fat on them without it being called fat or obese. Over time, however, these fat deposits can grow into more permanent fixtures on our bodies which become less and less accessible to the body to use as energy or fuel.

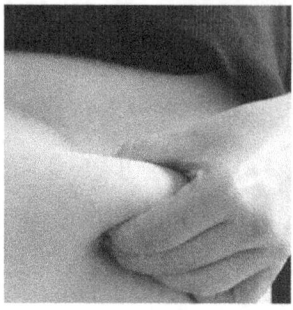 **Abnormal Reserves**

Just like the name states, abnormal fat is not normal. Abnormal fat builds up in the strangest and unflattering places. **Guys** usually get the 'Love Handles', 'Beer Guts' and 'Man Boobs'. **Women** suffer with 'Thunder Thighs', 'Muffin Top' and other sundry embarrassments. **Teens** can suffer from these very same problems.

As obesity progresses, you start to get extra fat deposits around internal organs such as the heart and lungs which can hamper their proper operation. For each **10 pounds of fat, the body builds 3 miles of blood vessels**. This is why obese people have high blood pressure, as the heart has to work extra hard to get blood through all these extra miles of vessels.

Abnormal fat is a potential source of fuel for the body, but unlike normal fat, it is not normally available to the body for energy. It has been **'locked away'** like in a safe deposit box, without a key to get at it!

Even in starvation mode, abnormal fat is utilized only after all other energy sources are used up. This is why on other weight loss programs the body will burn lean body mass *(mostly muscle)* before it gets to the abnormal fat reserves.

*I think the following by **Erma Bombeck** is funny and had become exactly how I felt.*

It is my theory you

can't lose fat.

All you do is move it

around like furniture.

If nothing ever changed, there would be no butterflies.

We all have big changes in our lives that are more or less a second chance.

~ Harrison Ford

All changes, even the most longed for have their melancholy;

For what we leave behind us is a part of ourselves;

We must die to one life before we can enter another.

~ Anatole France

Discovering Human Chorionic Gonadotropin (hCG)

You're probably wondering just want hCG can do for you. To begin with hCG stimulates the hypothalamus, which in turn begins **burning stored abnormal fat** at an average rate of 2500 calories per day. The amount of fat is released into the blood stream to be utilized as fuel by the body. Due to the fact that around 3500 calories of fat weighs about one pound, the result is **fat burned** and inches reduced! Some users report up to a pound or more per day of weight reduction when they begin the program.

Another wonderful effect that hCG has is that it reduces or eliminates hunger pangs in most people *(women, men or teen)*. hCG assists the hypothalamus in re-setting the metabolism in a number of ways. The hypothalamus gland controls fat storage, its utilization, hunger, and your metabolism as well as several other body functions as previously shown.

hCG is the match that lights the fire to adjust or re-set your metabolism.

Best Way to Benefit from hCG?

hCG By Prescription!

From my research and study, it's my belief that the true and authentic hCG is only by prescription. *I realize this can be very controversial, but after my research it's what I truly believe and recommend.*

hCG has not been approved nor is it controlled by the FDA as a treatment for obesity. This is caused most specifically by the FDA's immovability in classifying obesity as a condition that could be treatable.

In order to get the real injectable hCG, a physician will need to prescribe it for you. Due to this requirement, some people have resorted to purchasing the substances from foreign suppliers, like China or India, with a USA address. *I do not recommend taking this course of action, because no one can be entirely sure of the purity or source of such a product!*

Also due to current popularity of hCG it has come out that much of the hCG being sold on the 'so called black or underground market' is derived from animals and being imported into various countries *(including the USA)* from places such as China and India, again being sent from USA addresses.

Homeopathic hCG For Weight Control

Controversy and **erroneous** information about and shortages of the true injectable hCG for weight loss have led to substantial internet promotion of 'homeopathic hCG' and other forms for weight control. *If prepared by the true homeopathic dilution, then the homeopathic hCG would contain only a trace amount of real hCG.* **I would also question the source of the hCG.** *(FYI: Every manufacturer receives a mandatory data sheet showing the source of the ingredient they purchase. Ask to receive a printed copy of it).* These preparations are generally advertised for oral use only. Could this indicate the hCG has **not** been purified enough to be injectable?

Proponents of injected hCG for weight control have objected to homeopathic hCG as ineffective. Yet some people use it and are satisfied, at least temporarily.

Other types of hCG

You will find in the market place, especially over the internet all types of hCG drops, sprays or sublingual pills that claim to do exactly what the original Dr. Simeons hCG did. Many have proven to be nothing except an inert liquid and others have been found to contain some hCG greatly diluted and could be mixed with other ingredients. Price of those products could be a factor, but then maybe not. For myself, I would be skeptical about the products and not waste my money or time . . . or hope by using them.

You don't need a doctor's prescription to obtain them. But you never know just where they came from and who did the mixing or how sterile or safe they are.

In the summer of 2009 there was a brief story on TV

done by an investigative news reporter, airing in Salt Lake City. An undercover reporter called a number advertising the sale of hCG. The reporter made the arrangement to meet a woman at a designated location and was given a description to identify the car that the woman said she would be driving. When the reporter approached, the woman got out of her car, introducing herself to the reporter.

She then proceeded to open the trunk of her car and took out two containers, then walked to the hood of her car and began mixing a white powder that was purported to be hCG *(?)*, then mixing it with a liquid *(water?)*. She put both ingredients into a dropper bottle shaking it vigorously. She then handed the bottle to the reporter in exchange for cash. *(Due to an interruption, I don't recall the price the reporter paid for the bottle or if the price was ever mentioned)*.

This was in the heat of the summer and you should be aware that hCG **must** be kept in a cool place at all times, especially after it is mixed. Of course if the product was inert *(not good)*, it wouldn't matter would it? What did the reporter get? I don't know.

I only offer this as a word of caution. You usually get exactly what you pay for. The true, pure active hGC is not cheap, so be cautious if you are serious about your health and burning up your fat.

What I Have Observed

It seems that those who use the oral drops, spray or pill form of hCG don't stabilize their weight as quickly, nor keep it off as well as those who administer the hCG by injection, as recommended by Dr. Simeons.

Freedom of choice of the mind and spirit is God given ... Freedom from tyranny must be fought for and won.

~ Luci Flint

My Choice

I Decided to use Injectable hCG plus Vitamin B12

My doctor prescribed Vitamin B12 to be mixed with the hCG (*½ to ½*). I was grateful for the prescription. From my research, I believe B12 is critically important because the research says that most everyone is deficient in Vitamin B12. *(Look it up on the internet.)*

This being true, is it any wonder that there is an epidemic of 'nerve problems' such as anxiety, depression, anger, fear and the whole variety of nerve problems regulated primarily by the hypothalamus.

Why? It's my belief that the main reason so many are deficient of B12 is due to their eating and drinking habits. Vitamin B12 is easily destroyed by even mild acids such as naturally occurring gastric acid, which is one of the main secretions of the stomach and consists mainly of h**ydrochloric acid** that acidifies the stomach content to a pH of 1 to 2. Also due to the acidity of Vitamin C *(even the buffered type)* when taken with the B vitamins and especially B12, is much too acid, thus destroying the B's.

When you take a multi-B Complex tablet you should always take it with a meal and maybe even a little milk. This helps dilute the extreme acidity of your stomach. Never take it at the same time you take a Vitamin C supplement.

To receive the full benefit of B12 it must be taken either as a sub-lingual tablet dissolved under the tongue *(never chewed)* **or** via an injection. There is also a spray, which I tried once but felt I didn't get the benefit I should have from its use.

My instructions were to give myself an injection of hCG + Vitamin B12 *(both are included in the same injection)* every day for 40 days. Since I had administered injections previously to myself and others, I choose that method as it seemed the best way for the body to quickly utilize and benefit from both the B12 and hCG. Also it was the part of the protocol developed by Dr Simeons and I wanted to follow his as closely as possible.

With the decision made to use the injectable hCG

mixed with Vitamin B12, I was anxious to begin. When I arrived back home with my hCG and Vitamin B12 and the needles, I immediately sat down and **filled all** the needles with the hCG and B12, then put them in a baggie and in the fridge ready to use each day.

I administered the injection into my thigh, switching sides each day. There was no chance of the injection hurting as I figured my thighs were amply supplied with fat. But really the needle is so small *(like the needles used by a diabetic)* you virtually feel nothing. I always cleaned the injection area with an alcohol swab before administering it.

Having done the research and knowing the physiology of the body I felt that my system could become too accustom to a product like the hCG. Instead of giving me an injection daily for 40 days as previously instructed by my doctor, **I gave myself an injection each morning for six days, but NOT on the seventh day.** I felt this was important to give my body/system a one day of rest so it possibly wouldn't become immune to the benefits of the hCG. *(That is why in other places in the book I refer to my protocol time of*

40+ days).

(FYI: I started my Phase 1 of the protocol by giving myself an hCG shot on Monday through Saturday. **No injection on Sunday,** *which made it easy for me to keep on track).*

The hardest thing to learn in life is
Which bridge to cross and
Which bridge to burn . . .

~ David Russell

Using the power of decision gives you the capacity to get past any excuse to change any and every part of your Life in an instant.

~ Anthony Robbins

Slim and Shapely ~ Your Body

Yes, You Can Re-Shape it with hCG plus Nutrition

I know this is the section that you have been waiting for. I know you've been wondering what you could eat for only 500 calories a day and be satisfied, haven't you?

If you eat healthy foods, your cellular processes will work normally. But if you drink sodas and eat bad foods *(i.e. those that are man-made, processed, chemically treated or cooked wrong)* you will find your cellular processes will break down from lack of proper nutrition. Your cell structure will become impaired and have to work harder to compensate. When this happens, unfortunately, diseases can and do occur.

Healthy eating also helps keep the body balanced. Hormone production is normal. Muscle building occurs at a normal rate and **fat burning** occurs. The vitamins, minerals, enzymes and amino acids your body consumes are activated, absorbed and used for energy regulation.

Why we don't eat properly

There are various reasons why we don't eat nutritious foods. Here are a couple of the more common excuses:

- "Eating right is hard to do because the stores sell foods that are ready to eat. I know they are processed, have preservatives and all that, but they are so quick and easy. Besides I'm too exhausted to do anything else!"

- "I just flat don't have time. I've got to be at such and such meeting; or I have to get three different kids to three different places at the same time. One has to get to baseball practice; one to dance class; and one to the piano teacher. How could anyone even expect me to go shopping, cook and serve a meal, when I have all that to do? Why shouldn't I just pick up something at the drive-in and be done with it? It's so much easier and the kids love it."

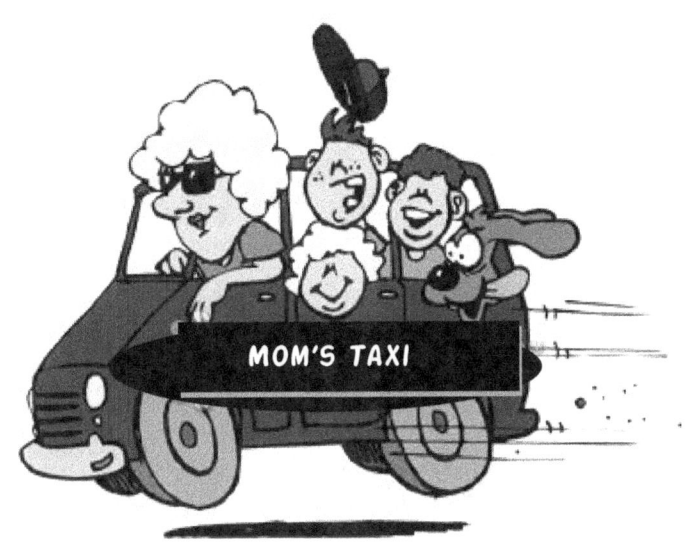

SOMETIMES IT IS NOT ENOUGH TO DO OUR BEST WE MUST DO WHAT IS REQUIRED

~ *Sir* Winston Churchill

TRUST YOURSELF AS YOU REALLY KNOW MORE THAN YOU THINK YOU DO~

~ Luci Flint

Eating Protocol

What You Will Eat While Taking hCG

The rules are really simple. Some would say that they are absolutely boring.

If you feel that way, know it's up to you to 'spice up' your meals and still stay on track. I'll give a few hints on what I did that made it a lot easier and more appetizing. I love good tasting, attractively served food. That is why I enjoy gourmet cooking . . . yet this is anything but gourmet cooking.

After shopping I would weigh all my meats and veggies, before putting them up. Most of the meat I froze, and the veggies I put in individual baggies ready to steam while I cooked my meat. I was extremely busy at that time so I would actually prepare most of my food for the week on Saturday. I also had my husband to think about and he didn't need to burn fat. I planned and cooked him nutritious meals, which were similar to mine, but substantially more.

You will begin your hCG protocol with three **actions** and **two phases.**

The very **first actions** are for you to:

1) Measure yourself   and   2) Weigh yourself

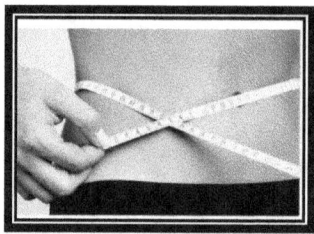 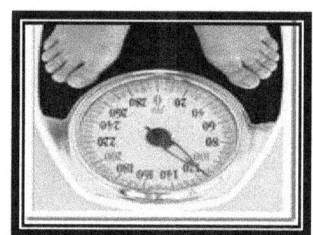

Now is the time when you take off all your clothes to take your measurements and weigh yourself. *(I know . . . you hope no one is peeking).*

Here is what you need to do: Write down all your measurements and weight. I used a spiral notepad for my records, keeping it near the scales. I also recorded any thoughts or reactions I experienced. You will be weighing daily and measuring yourself approximately every two weeks.

Here is your measurement list

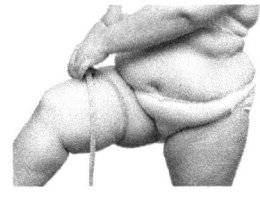

(No, this is not a picture of me)!

For Men, Teens, and Women

- *Upper chest (under arm pits above breast)*

- *Rib cage (nipple level – women to include the breast)*

- *Waist (approximately the level of the belly button)*

- *Hips (5" below your waist)*

- *Buttocks (largest part of your hips)*

- *Both thighs, knees, calves, ankles (separately)*

- *Both upper arms, elbows, wrists (separately)*

Every two weeks you will add up all the inches you reduced *(taking your beginning measurement and subtracting the last measurement . . . this will be the inches you have reduced in that particular area. Then total all the inches you've reduced. I believe you'll be shocked, but extremely pleased too. I know I was)!*

Action 3: Within this book you have a list of foods,

drinks and other suggestions. Make a list or take the book with you and venture to the store. Get as much and as many items you can afford. This way you won't have to go to the store that often or be tempted to buy things you shouldn't have. Too, you'll have them on hand for easy access and not have any excuses as to why you didn't stay on track with your diet. *(See under **Free Offer** page 143 for information on what brands I found the best and highly recommend).*

Phase 1: Loading On Days 1 & 2 + hCG Injections

As I said previously there are **two important phases** for your hCG protocol. The **first phase** is what is called **loading days**. After taking your measurements and weight, immediately give yourself your first hCG injection. Look at the time as you will want to keep as close to that time scheduled each morning for your injection. (*If for some reason you miss that exact time, **do not skip** your injection. Take it the minute you can. A day skipped can be days lost without weight reduction).* After the injection you must initialize the rest of the protocol by **eating excessively for the first 2 days** - solid.

This is not a joke. There is good reason to do this. During the first 2 days you need to eat as much as possible of all kinds of foods to the point of being past full. If you aren't hungry, eat anyway. If you don't feel like having another sandwich, eat it anyway. Healthy food would be nice, but not required during this phase.

Remember you will take your hCG injection every morning starting with . . . Phase 1 – Day 1

Loading properly prepares you for the next phase of the **500 Calorie Diet**. If you do not **load** properly you will have a much slower start and may suffer with hunger pangs.

Phase 2: 3rd Day and Forward begins your 500 Calorie Diet plus hGC Injection

On your hCG protocol, you can eat your meals **two or three times** during the day, it's your choice. You can have **two snack times only**, one mid-morning **or** mid-afternoon and one just before going to bed. Whatever you decide **you are to consume no more than a total of 500 calories per day.** Since the body normally uses around 2500 calories per day the hypothalamus will use the 500 calories from your meals and take the rest of what it needs from your abnormal fat.

If you have prepared yourself properly during the **loading** phase the hCG will reduce or eliminate your hunger. Impulse eaters must apply **will power** against any psychological urges to eat and must fight off cravings.

Since the hypothalamus is 'dumping' fat into your blood stream, you must drink at least 1/2 gallon *(64 ounces or 2 liters)* of water per day - more is preferable. Actually you should at least drink one-half of your body weight in ounces. *Example: If you weigh 200 pounds (91 kilos or 14.3 stone), you should drink 100 ounces (3 liters) of water per day.* Drinking water is one of the ways to flush the fat out of your body. **Do not drink** carbonated water or other flavored waters or drinks, soda pop, tea, coffee, or liquor and count them **as part** of your water intake. They will not wash the fat out of your system properly and will change the pH of your blood chemistry, dramatically slowing any fat burning.

500 Calories a Day is More Than You Think!

*This begins on the **third day** after two days of **loading** as previously revealed.*

First began each day with the **fresh juice of 1 lemon or lime** in a glass or cup of hot or cold water. If desired add a few drops of Stevia to sweeten. (*I purchased Stevia at the health food store. I understand that it is now in most grocery stores - read labels before purchasing*).

Breakfast:

Six days of the week:

*(**Remember hCG injections for 6 days**)*

Fruit: Days 1 – 3 - 5

- **Strawberries** *(3 oz or 85 grams – these can be sliced and sweetened with Stevia if desired. Sometimes I poured Walden Farms Chocolate Syrup over my berries. If I ate them whole, I dipped them in Walden Farms Chocolate Dip. Learn more about this later).*

- **Melba toast** *(1 round only)*

Days 2 – 4 - 6

Eat one-half of a Pink Grapefruit . . . OR one-half of a Cantaloupe.

Special Note: Some medications advise you not to eat grapefruit. If so **Do Not Eat It**. Eat strawberries or cantaloupe instead or use the egg recipe below.

Day 7 have the following (*No hCG injection today***).**

• **Scramble 1 whole egg, mixed with the whites of two eggs.** *(Salsa that has only 5 calories per 1 tablespoon is delightful with your eggs).*

• **Melba toast** *(1 round only)*

DON'T FORGET TO DRINK YOUR WATER~

Lunch: 1 Protein plus 1 Vegetable only

Protein: *(All visible fat must be removed before cooking. You must weigh the meat while it is **raw**. You can have 3 ounces or 85 grams of **protein twice a day**).*

All protein must be broiled or grilled without additional fat. Should you need just a smidgen of fat, you can use one-half teaspoon of organic, cold-pressed virgin **coconut oil**, which has medium chain triglycerides *(MCT)* that does not convert to fat as most other oils do. You can also use no-calorie salad dressing or Bragg's Liquid Aminos spray.

*(Walden Farms has a great variety of salad dressing, plus there are such items as **BBQ Sauce**, both the **Thick & Spicy** and the **Hickory Smoked; Seafood Sauce; Ketchup; Mayo** and **Mustard** and much more. All their products have **no fats, sugars or calories** . . . yet are surprisingly delicious with no after taste. They do not interfere with the fat burning or reduction of weight or inches. If the local health food or specialty stores don't carry Walden Farms products, you can log onto their website: **http://www.waldenfarms.com.** They are exceptionally accommodating and will send the products directly to you. I purchase **Bragg's Liquid Aminos Spray** at the health food store.)*

Meats you can eat

- Burger *(very lean)*

- Beef *(very lean)*

- Chicken Breast *(skinless)*

- Crab *(real – not imitation)*

- White Fish *(Fresh or Frozen)*

- Lobster *(Fresh or Frozen)*

- Shrimp *(Fresh or Frozen)*

- Tilapia *(Fresh or Frozen)*

- Veal

(All frozen products must be thawed and weighed before cooking).

Do Not Eat The Following:

- Dried or pickled fish

- Eel

- Herring

- Roasts

- Salmon

- Sardines *(fresh or canned)*

- Tuna *(fresh or canned)*

Vegetable: Only **one** type of vegetable is eaten per meal (*i.e. 3 oz or 85 grams –do not mix vegetables; the* *one exception is you can have mixed salad greens).*

- Asparagus

- Beet greens

- Cabbage

- Celery

- Chard

- Chicory

- Cucumbers

- Fennel

- Green Salad *(Organic Mixed Greens)*

- Onions

- Red Radishes

- Tomatoes

Carbs: 1 Melba toast OR 1 Grissino breadstick at a time, with either your meal or with your fruit as a snack. *(i.e. **Never** eat both fruits and breads at the same time). P.S. Melba toast or Grissino are only 5 calories each and not considered as bread, so to speak.*

Fruits That Are Allowed To Be Eaten:

You are allowed only **two fruits portions per day**. *(i.e. This could be one large apple, **not two small apples**; ½ pink grapefruit, or ½ cantaloupe, which equals one portion).*

- Apple

- Cantaloupe

- Grapefruit *(½ - pink)*

- Lemons *(unlimited)*

- Limes *(unlimited)*

- Strawberries *(3 oz or 105 gm)*

KEEP DRINKING YOUR WATER~

Dinner:

Choices are the same as for lunch. Try changing **them up** a little so you don't get bored with your meals. Variety not only makes your meals more appealing, but variety also gives you different nutrients during the day.

Snacks:

You can use your fruit for a snack in the mid-morning **or** mid-afternoon **or** for a bedtime snack, along with one piece of Melba toast or Grissino breadstick, **if you haven't consumed them at another meal**.

I liked to eat my apple with one piece of Melba toast while relaxing with a hot cup of chamomile tea, sweetened lightly with Stevia before going to bed.

First Few Days

On the day after the third injection it is routine to hear these remarks:

• "You know, I'm sure it's only psychological, but I already feel quite different".

• "Now that I have been allowed to eat anything I want, I can't seem to get it down. Since yesterday I feel like a stuffed pig. Food just doesn't seem to interest me anymore and I am longing to really get on with my diet".

• "I noticed that I seemed to be passing more urine and

the swelling in my ankles has really gone down since I started dieting and taking my hCG injections."

Many of you might find the same thing. That's great! It means you are shedding the excess water in your tissue.

By the fourth day you should be feeling fine and you will settle down in your thinking and just start to enjoy the diet as you see a continuous reduction in inches and weight.

Important Notice: Some people have a buildup of internal toxins before they start their hCG diet. Some will complain of a headache. Know that it is not uncommon for this to happen. It is alright to take an aspirin for your headache, but don't overdo aspirin as it could affect your hypothalamus. After all **aspirin is a drug**.

It is usually at this point that a difference appears between those people who have literally eaten to capacity *(loading)* during the first two days of the hCG injections and those who have not. The former feel remarkably well, they have no hunger, nor do they feel tempted when others eat normally at the same table. They feel lighter, more clear-headed and notice a desire to move, quite contrary to their previous lethargy.

Those who have **disregarded** the advice to eat to capacity *(loading)* continue to have minor discomforts and do not have the same euphoric sense of self-being until a week or so later. It seems that their normal fat reserves require that much more time before they are fully stocked.

Making up the Calories

The diet used in conjunction with hCG must not exceed 500 calories per day! The way these calories are made up is of utmost importance. For instance if you drop the apple and eat an extra breadstick instead, you will not be getting more calories but **you will not reduce your weight**. There are a number of foods particularly fruits and vegetables, which have the same or even lower caloric values than those listed as permissible and yet we find that **they interfere** with the regular **burning of the fat** to reduce your weight under hCG, presumably owing to the nature of their composition. Examples of forbidden items are:

- Artichokes
- Carrots
- Pears
- Peppers
- Pimiento
- And many others ~ *just stick with the diet.*

Faulty Dieting

A few of you will take my word that the slightest deviation from the diet can have **disastrous results** as far as the weight is concerned. This extreme sensitivity has the advantage that the smallest error is immediately detectable at your daily weighing. Yet many have to experience it before you really believe it.

Your Job Can Make a Difference

If your job is in a high official position such as embassy personnel, politician, senior executive, etc., where you are obliged to attend social functions to which you cannot bring your meager meal you must know and understand that an official dinner will cost you the loss of about three days of weight reduction, regardless of how careful you are and in spite of a friendly and would-be cooperative host.

I suggest you avoid any embarrassment by avoiding the almost inevitable turn of conversation to your weight problem and the outpouring of lay counsel from your table partners by **not letting it be known** that your **are** on a special diet.

You should take dainty servings of everything, hide what you can under the cutlery and under your napkin when you are finished eating. Forego the liquor toasts *(toast with your water instead),* forget the bread and butter, crackers, etc. regardless of how tempting they look. If soup is served, act as if you are taking a dip or two touching your lips, but **not** putting it into your mouth. If the salad already has dressing on, either dig in where it might not have any or forgo eating it. **Absolutely don't eat the dessert.**

You must realize any weight gain may take two to three days to get rid of. But that is one of the sacrifices which your profession entails. Allowing three days for your correction of such incidents do not jeopardize your scheduled plan provided they do not occur all too frequently. If this is your case maybe it would be better if you postponed your diet to a socially more peaceful *(less busy)* season.

Vitamins and Anemia

Sooner or later most of you will express a fear that you may be running out of vitamins or that the restricted diet may make you anemic. On this score you should be confidently relieved of this apprehension by understanding every time **you burn** a pound of fatty tissue, which you do almost daily with only the actual **fat burned.** The foods that contain the vitamins, minerals, enzymes and proteins, get circulated in your blood and are in abundance to feed back into your body. Actually, a low blood count not due to any serious disorder of the blood forming tissues improves during your hCG injections and 500 calorie diet. In studies it has never been noted or encountered of a significant protein deficiency or signs of a lack of vitamins when you are doing you prescribed hCG protocol.

Just a quick note . . . if you previously took nutritional supplements and they did not contain enzymes in the formula you wasted your money. You need to know that for the body to utilize the nutrition they must contain: (1) multiple vitamins, which require; (2) minerals and minerals require (3) enzymes. Without those three things you might as well flush your money down the toilet because that is where you supplements end up, so you actually receive little or no value.

Fluctuations in Weight Reduction
Men vs Women

After the fourth or fifth day of dieting the daily reduction of weight begins to decrease to one pound or somewhat less per day, and there is a smaller urinary output.

Men often continue to lose regularly at that rate. Women are more irregular **in spite of faultless dieting**. There may be no drop at all for two or three days and then a sudden loss which re-establishes the normal average. These fluctuations are entirely due to variations in the retention and elimination of water, which are more marked in women than in men.

The weight registered by the scales is determined by

two processes, not necessarily synchronized under the influence of hCG. Fat is being extracted from the cells and stored in the fatty tissue. When these cells are empty and therefore serve no purpose, the body breaks down the cellular structure and absorbs it by breaking up of the useless cells, connective tissue, blood vessels, etc. This could cause a lag in the process of fat-extraction. When this happens the body appears to replace some of the extracted fat with water which is retained for this purpose. As water is heavier than fat the scales may show no reduction of weight although sufficient fat has actually been burned up and this is where the inches can make a difference in your overall reduction. When such tissue is finally broken down the water is liberated and there is a sudden flood of urine and a marked reduction of weight.

This is a simple interpretation of what is really an extremely complex mechanism that you should understand when on the hCG diet. This is why you need to know that on certain days you do not lose,

An interesting feature of the hCG method is that regardless of how much abnormal fat you have the greatest circumference -- abdomen or hips as the case may be is reduced at a constant rate.

Women Only ~ Menstrual Interruption
(Men need to understand this too)

Those of you, who are still in this period of your life, need to know that interruption in weight reduction could often occur a few days before and during the menstrual period and with some women at the time of ovulation.

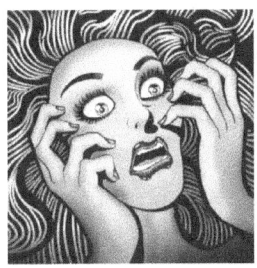

Diet Errors - Be Aware

Any interruption of the normal weight reduction is always due to some possibly very minor dietary error. Similarly, any gain of more than a half a pound is invariably the result of some transgression or mistake unless it happens on or about the day of ovulation or during the three days preceding the onset of menstruation in which case it should be ignored. In all other cases the reason for the gain must be established at once.

If you admit that you had stepped out of your hCG diet protocol when you see that you are not reducing as you think you should, you might not have realized some of the following slipups:

You might be surprised because unless you know and remember that your lack of weight reduction could be caused by these simple little thoughtless acts:

- One salted almond, or a couple of salted peanuts

- A couple of potato chips

- A small glass of tomato juice

- An orange

I know it's hard to believe that such small things will bring about a definite increase in your weight on the following day.

You might wonder why extra food weighing only one ounce should increase your weight by six

ounces. You need to understand the following:

Under the influence of hCG the blood is saturated with food and the blood volume has adapted itself so that it can only accommodate the 500 calories which come from the intestinal tract during the course of the day. Any additional calories, however little they may be cannot be accommodated and the blood is therefore forced to increase its volume sufficiently to hold the extra food, which it can only do in a much diluted form *(water retention)*. Thus it is not the weight of what is eaten that plays the determining role but rather the amount of water which the body must retain to accommodate the forbidden food or drink.

This can be illustrated by mentioning the case of salt. In order to hold **one teaspoonful of salt the body requires one liter** *(34 ounces)* **of water** as it cannot accommodate salt in any higher concentration. Thus, if you consume what is equal to one teaspoonful of salt your weight will go up by more than two pounds as soon as this salt is absorbed from your intestine into your blood.

To this explanation you might ask the question: "Well,

if I put on that much every time I eat a little extra, how I can hold my weight after the treatment?" **It must therefore be made clear that this only happens as long as you are taking hCG.** When you are over your program the blood is no longer saturated and can easily accommodate extra food without having to increase its volume. Here again you need to know that this interpretation is a simplification of an extremely intricate physiological process which actually accounts for the phenomenon.

Salt and Reducing

While I'm on the subject of salt I want to take this opportunity to explain that there is no restriction in the use of salt . . . but **you must drink** large quantities of water throughout the hCG protocol.

You are out to reduce your **abnormal fat** and should not in the least be concerned or interested in such illusory weight reduction that could be achieved by depriving the body of salt, which could desiccate the body. Though you are allowed the free use of salt the daily amount taken should be roughly the same. A sudden increase of salt will of course be followed by a corresponding increase in weight as shown by the scale. An increase in the intake of salt is one of the most common causes for an increase in weight from one day to the next. Such an increase can be ignored provided it is accounted for. It in no way influences the regular burning of your fat.

Water – Water – Water

Far too many people are hard to convince that the amount of water they retain has nothing to do with the amount of water they drink. When your body is forced to retain water it will do so at all costs. If the fluid intake is insufficient to provide all the water required, your body withholds water from the kidneys and your urine becomes scanty and highly concentrated. This imposes a certain strain on the kidneys. If your fluid is insufficient, excessive water will be with-drawn from the intestinal tract with the result that the feces become hard and dry. On the other hand if you drink more than your body requires the surplus is promptly and easily eliminated. Trying to prevent the body from retaining water by drinking less is therefore not only futile but even harmful and dangerous.

Constipation

An excess of water keeps feces soft, which is very important to the obese who commonly suffer from constipation and a spastic colon. When taking hCG and on the 500 calorie diet you should **never use any kind of laxative taken by mouth**. You should know that owing to the restricted diet it is perfectly satisfactory and normal to have an evacuation of the bowel only once every two or three days. If plenty of fluids are taken the slight constipation never leads to any great disturbance. If you are still constipated you might need to increase your intake of water until you return to normal by having **elimination daily**. With my **Free Offer** *(on page 143)* you'll learn more about how to prevent constipation.

My failures have been errors

in judgment, not of intent.

~ Ulysses S. Grant

Inevitable Plateau

Yes, even with hCG you most likely will hit a plateau. When a plateau happens you have one choice to break the plateau:

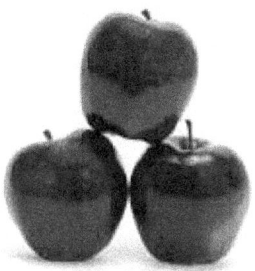

Your Choice:

Have an 'Apple Day'

How do you know if you've hit a plateau? Only if you find that you have **not** reduced in weight or inches for three days. Then there is only one choice when this happens and one I highly recommend . . . an **Apple Day.** You'll be surprised how easy and filling this Apple Day can be I know I was. In fact I was never able to eat more than three medium size apples. I've heard other say they could barely get four eaten. However, you can eat as many as you want.

*Understand you will **eat nothing** else but **Apples** and **drink water** for the entire day. No Melba toast or Grissino breadstick.*

I can tell you that I got more done on my Apple Day because I didn't have to stop and eat. Because of my writing I just munched apples, drank lots of water and kept on writing.

You'll find that the Apple Day can jog your metabolism to begin burning fat again.

The 3 Day Rule

I remember on the 15th day of the diet I thought I had hit a plateau. However I was determined to go the **three days** before trying anything else so I ate as usual. My surprise was on the third day I lost 5 pounds. Wow, that was exciting! It was on my 27th day before I actually hit a plateau and the Apple Day did the trick.

Remember everyone's metabolism is different so only your watchful eye; weighing yourself and measuring for inches reduced in your major areas will tell you if you are on a plateau.

*P.S. Sometimes I liked to dip my apples in either **Carmel Dip** or **Chocolate Dip** made by **Walden Farms**. Their delicious dips add no calories, and don't interfere with the protocol and are a delightful alternative to just plain foods, even apples and strawberries).*

And YES, you continue to take your hCG injection on your Apple Day, unless it is the 7th day.

Life is not about finding yourself
Life is about creating yourself!

Life is not about waiting for the storms to pass

It is about learning how to

Dance in the Rain!

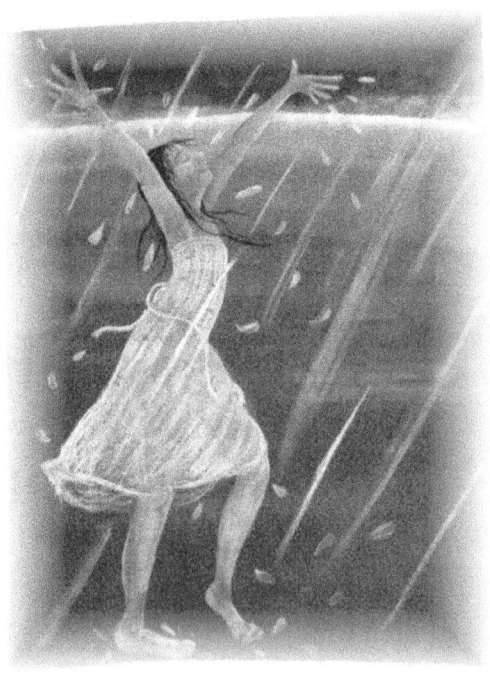

Weight Stabilization

You and the Scales

You must weigh yourself every morning when you get out of bed. **First empty your bladder** then strip off your clothes and weigh yourself just before you shower.

You must <u>continue</u> 3 days on the 500 calorie diet after you have taken <u>all</u> your injections. It <u>takes 3 weeks after the end of the hCG injections and protocol for your weight to stabilize.</u> *(i.e. the scale does not show violent fluctuations after an occasional excess).* During this period you must realize that the carbohydrates that convert to glucose *(sugars)*, regular sugar, or even honey that you eat along with, white rice, bread, potatoes, pastries etc, are by far the most dangerous. If no carbohydrates whatsoever are eaten, fats can be indulged in somewhat more liberally. In other words don't eat carbs and sweets at the same meal, if at all. **As soon as fats and starch *(carbs)* are combined things are very liable to get out of hand.** This has to be observed very carefully especially during the **first 3 weeks <u>after</u> the hCG protocol is ended**. Otherwise disappointments are almost sure to occur in unwanted pounds and inches.

Skipping a Meal

As long as your weight stays within two pounds of the weight reached on the **day of your last injection** you should take no notice of any increase. But the moment the scale goes beyond two pounds or 1 kilo, even if it is only a few ounces **you must on that same day entirely skip breakfast and lunch, drinking plenty of water. In the evening you must eat a huge steak with only one apple OR one raw tomato.** Of course this rule applies only to your morning weight. Previously obese people should never check their weight during the day as there may be wide fluctuations and these are merely alarming and confusing.

It is **critically important** that the meal skipped is on the **same day the scale registers an increase of more than two pounds or 1 kilo and that meal is not postponed until the following day.** Skipping of the meal . . . and **skipping means literally not eating**

anything, not just having a light meal but following the above suggestion. **If this action is postponed the phenomenon does not occur** and several days of strict dieting may be necessary to correct the situation. I found that I hardly ever needed to skip a meal.

3 Days after You Finish Taking hCG

After you finish taking the hCG injections, you will stay on the 500 Calorie Diet for three days, while you body adjusts. After that you start back on a semi-regular diet. I suggest you keep as close to 1000 calories per day as possible.

I have noted that if I'd eaten a fairly heavy lunch I felt no desire to eat dinner and in this case I had no weight increase. If I keep my weight at the point reached at the end of the protocol even a heavy dinner once in a while does not bring about an increase of weight the next morning and therefore does not call for any special measures.

Like most others that have been on the hCG diet you will be surprised how small your appetite has become and yet how much you can eat without gaining weight.

You no longer suffer from an abnormal appetite and feel satisfied with much less food than before.

FYI . . . If you still need to reduce your weight after the 40+ day protocol . . . you will have to wait six weeks before beginning again. But this time will be much easier, because you know the protocol and what to expect.

Discipline is the

bridge between

Goals and

Accomplishments. "

~ *Jim Rohn*

Concluding Your Diet

Again, this is very important. You must remember to continue **three days on the 500 calorie diet after your last injection.** After that you can begin eating other foods. Try to stay on about 1000 calories a day.

I know I've repeated numerous points throughout the book. I did so to emphasis how critical and important those suggestions are.

May I suggest something else to you? Take out one of your old pictures of when **you were fat**. Remember how you ate before starting you hCG diet? Don't fall back into your old habits. It might be helpful to review your '40 days' list you made in the beginning where you wrote down all the foods you ate and things you drank. Review them so you don't make the same mistakes. *(Now put the picture away . . . as you don't want to keep that image before you or think about it all the time)*

Remember so as you thinketh . . . so as you become!

~Luci Flint

Rule: Don't mix carbs and sugars together at the same time! Always remember to eliminate as much sugar and carbs *(pasta, breads, pastries, potatoes and white rice, etc.)* as much as possible.

You must continue to weigh yourself. If you see you've gained some extra pounds and they remain after 4 or 5 days *(no longer than ten days should go by before you make adjustments)*, you will know you need to re-adjust your diet to reduce back down to your ideal weight. Try an Apple Day **or** you might try a day where you skip breakfast and lunch, and for dinner have a big delicious steak and one apple **or** one raw tomato, but not both. That is all . . . nothing else other than water.

Secret Revealed!

P.S. I'm sure you would like to 'indulge' once in a while to satisfy your **sweet tooth**. I don't blame you. I enjoy those goodies too. So here's the secret of eating your sweet things . . . **eat them between meals**, not with a meal of carbs, fats, and proteins. *(You should wait at least 90 minutes after you've eaten your meal or 90 minutes before eating a meal).*

EXERCISE

Last But Not Least

Many of you might have noticed that I didn't talk much about exercise and there is a reason. My much biased reason is that I believe that some people exercise too much and to their own determent.

When I lived in Dallas, Texas, I well remember the day that Jim Fixx, the 'running guru' dropped dead from heart failure while running on the track at the Aerobic Center. Here was a man who supposedly was in tip-top shape, without an ounce of extra fat. He wasn't all that old either; in fact if I remember right he was only in his mid to late forties. How could that have happened?

I do have an explanation, but won't go into the medical reason for cause of his possible demise in this book. *(It does however have to do with food and liquid consumption and the pH of the blood).* I mention it only because I believe he was perhaps excessive in his exercise program. *(I know I've read of other cases, but I don't remember them all . . . been too many and I don't want to take the time to search them out).*

Your Personalized Exercise

If you **have not** been into a regular exercise regimen, and decide to begin your exercise when beginning your hCG and 500 calorie diet protocol you might find it very difficult. I suggest you **don't start** a **vigorous** program at this time. I believe it could be a **serious mistake**.

Only if you've been an exercise buff **before** beginning the hCG regimen should you continue. Even then, it might be better and more beneficial if you curtail your most **vigorous** exercises during this period.

I encourage you to walk at a pace that you are comfortable with and gradually increase the distance of the walk. You should alter your speed a few times during your walk. Speed up for a pace or so, then slow back down. This adjusts the heart rate and seems to burn more fat than staying at a steady pace as it keeps giving a jump start to your metabolism. This is an exercise that most any one can do regardless of your age.

Dr. Al Sears, M.D. wrote an excellent book titled **'Pace'** *with the subtitle of* **'Discover Your Native Fitness'.** *You can buy the book over the internet.*

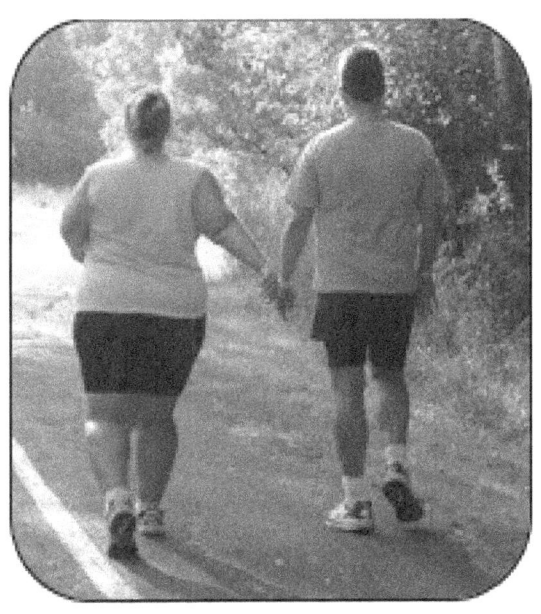

Riding a bike *(not a marathon)* is great exercise and again I suggest you pace yourself.

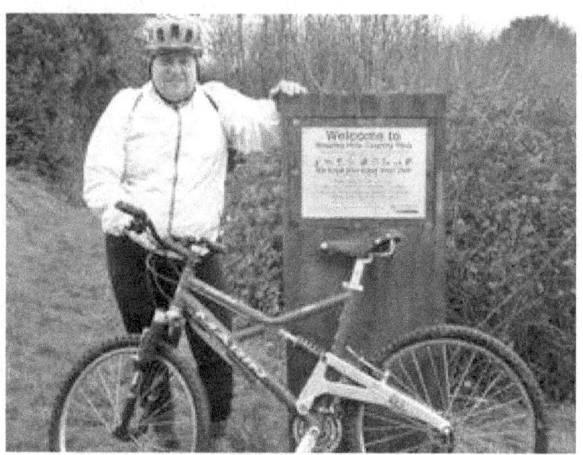

Swimming is also especially good as it exercises the entire body, which you can also pace. Just enjoy yourself while exercising.

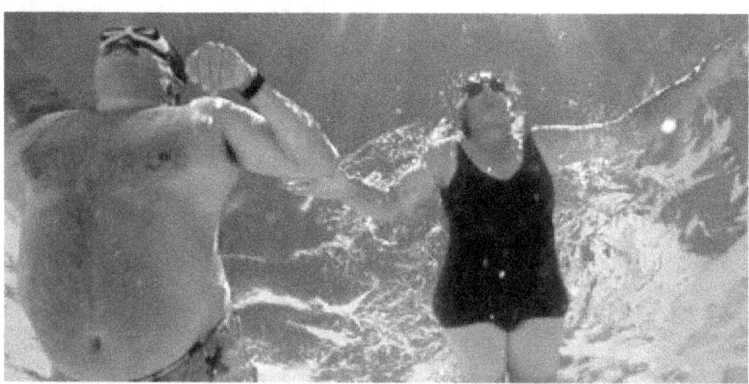

Help and Hints

The juice of one lemon or lime daily is allowed for all purposes. Other condiments you can use are salt, pepper, organic apple cider vinegar, mustard powder, garlic, sweet basil, parsley, thyme, marjoram, etc. and a small amount of coconut oil may be used for seasoning. **Absolutely no other oils, butter or dressings that contain calories, fat or sugars can be used!**

Herbal teas, coffee, and plain water are the only drinks allowed. However keep in mind that coffee and regular black or green tea, which both contain caffeine; or anything with caffeine can cause dehydration and could possibly alter the function of the hypothalamus, so go easy on them. They cannot be counted for the total intake of plain water. *(No liquor is allowed while on the protocol).*

As a reminder you **should drink at least one-half of your body weight in ounces per day in plain water**. Many people are afraid to drink so much water because they fear that this may make them retain more water. This is a wrong notion as the body is more inclined to store water when the intake falls below its normal requirements.

Snacks

The fruit and Melba toast or Grissino breadstick may be eaten between meals instead of with lunch or dinner. Remember **no more than two fruits** and **two pieces of** Melba toast **or** Grissino breadstick per day, but **never at the same time.**

Every item in your list of foods has been gone over carefully. I must **continually stress** the point that no variations other than those listed may be introduced. All things not listed are **forbidden** and you can be assured that nothing permissible has been left out. Always make sure the 3 oz or 85 grams of meat is scrupulously weighed raw after all visible fat has been removed. **All veggies must be weighed before cooking**. (*You'll be surprised how much 3 oz of mixed salad greens will be*).

It should also be mentioned that two small apples weighing as much as one large one **will not have the same caloric value** (*it will be higher*) **and therefore**

not allowed. Though there is no restriction on the size of **one apple**.

Some people do not realize that chicken breast **does not mean the breast of any other fowl** nor does it mean a wing or drumstick.

How to Weigh Your Food

To accurately weigh your food you must have the right type of scales. You need one that enables you to put a bowl or saucer on it, so you can then push the 'Tare' button which will take it back to zero. This allows you to measure your meat or veggie accurately. The brand I bought was a digital diet scale that was easy to read and had a flat glass disk to put a plate or bowl on. I purchased it at WalMart. But I'm sure you can pick them up at other places.

Too Much Food - 500 Calories?

There are a few people who feel that even so little food is too much for them, therefore they think they can omit anything they wish. But you must know it is best if you eat the 500 calories daily as it helps with the set-point and your metabolism to burn fat. There is no objection to breaking up you meals. For instance having a breadstick and an apple for breakfast or before going to bed, provided they are deducted from the regular meals.

The whole daily ration of two breadsticks or two fruits may **not be eaten at the same time**, nor can any item be saved from the previous day and then added on the following day.

In the beginning I suggest you do not rely on your memory for what you can eat. Check every meal against your approved list of food **before you eat**.

A Note of Warning

It is worth pointing out that **any attempt to observe this diet without hCG will lead to trouble in two to three days**. There have been cases in which people have proudly flaunted their dieting powers in front of their friends **without** mentioning the fact that they are also taking hCG. They let their friends try the 500 calorie diet and when this proves to be a failure - as it necessarily must - the person starts raking in unmerited kudos for superhuman willpower. This is not only wrong, it is dishonest.

Be truthful in all aspects – especially about your diet and hCG. I'm sure you don't want to cause what could be a serious situation with friends or loved ones.

If we are to go forward,

We must go back and

Rediscover those precious

Values that all reality

Hinges on moral foundations

And that all reality has spiritual control.

~ Martin Luther King, Jr.

Costs:

The price of the hCG depends on the physician you choose. I found their prices varied widely. So call around or get on the internet to search out sources. Then phone to interview different ones. Ask if they will send you via an email or fax *(if you have one)* a copy of their prices and protocol. An interview should go two-ways, not just the physician or his assistant. *(Caution . . .* **do not be tempted** *by some of the ads you'll see on the internet, billboards, or newspapers. There are many unscrupulous people and vendors out there and you might not get what you think you're paying for. Many just want your credit card number).*

Change does not roll in on the wheels of inevitability,

But comes through continuous struggles.

~ Martin Luther King, Jr.

Cosmetics

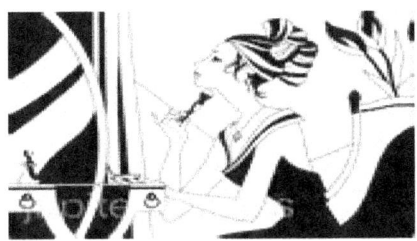

No Cosmetics - You've Got to Be Kidding~

Most women find it hard to believe that fats, oils, creams, and ointments applied to the skin are absorbed and interfere with hCG weight reduction just as if they had been eaten, but they really can!

When you burn a lot of fat there will be a natural occurring of sagging skin with more wrinkles and your skin may become quite dry. Most well meaning doctors or advisors will tell you that the only thing you can use on your skin is a little mineral oil. This myth keeps being perpetuated by the advisor or doctors, who just follow each other like sheep. **Please do not listen**

to that tripe.

Mineral oil is **addictive** to the skin and **does not allow your skin to breathe properly**. Yes, mineral oil is inert and isn't absorbed into the skin, but it is damaging to the skin. You'll probably end up with more wrinkles; skin that's dry and flaky; a marked increase in sagging skin, that is downright uncomfortable. You might have a slim body, but you might resemble an **old person** that looks like you have **thirty miles of bad road** from the appearance of wrinkles on your face and neck.

I hope you can find some product you can use. But you must to be very cautious and read the complete ingredient list. If you are unsure about some of the ingredients you can email me and I will answer your questions. See email address on page 134.

I was instructed by the doctor *(a plastic surgeon)* **not to use any cosmetics. Of course I didn't listen to his advice.** I know he is very knowledgeable, but I didn't believe he had the basic education in formulation of skin care and cosmetics in general. Since he was a plastic surgeon, who knows maybe he thought if I got wrinkled enough I would want a face lift.

(This was the 2nd time I didn't follow his instructions. The 1st time was when I made the decision to take the hCG for only 6 days and none on the 7th, instead of the continuous 40 days).

My Reasoning For Using Cosmetics

As a formulator, compounder, manufacturer and marketer of the first complete line of organic, botanical and active aloe vera cosmetics ever created; I knew that the doctor was dead wrong about using mineral oil or using no cosmetics.

I've been actively using and studying about Aloe Vera and other botanical oils and ingredients since 1958. Worldwide I'm known as **'the pioneer' of natural, botanical products. I'm also accredited as being the 'Mother of the Modern Aloe Vera Movement'.**

I have 100 formulas to my credit currently being marketed around the world. I first formulated them in 1970 and have used nothing on my face, body and hair since.

*I must tell you that at my current age of 75 (2010) I certainly didn't want my skin to become saggy and wrinkled. Most people can't believe I'm 75 and have **less wrinkles than I had at 35**. That is until I show them an unretouched photo of myself at 35 and a current unretouched photo or they see me in person They are always amazed by the texture and luminosity of my skin. And no, I've never had a surgical face lift, skin peel or Botox injections.*

No way can I go into that story in this 'diet book' but for those interested in learning more about how I've kept my youthful skin after losing 42 pounds *(19+ kilos or 3 stone – note that one stone is equal to 14 pounds)* email me at: **<u>Lucille@LucilleFlintFormulas.com</u>**

Before I continue on, please understand that I am NOT trying to sell you my cosmetic products. However, if you are sincere about wanting to know more about them, please contact me at the above email requesting more information specifically about my cosmetic formulas.

In fact, I strongly debated about putting in the following information. Yet my advisors, editor, and friends encouraged me to include the information. Knowing how hard it is to find products that can be used when on the hCG protocol without compromising it, I decided that it would be unfair to you and leave you hanging, so to speak.

How I Kept My Wrinkles Away?

Some of my formulations are extremely compatible without using oils that could interfere with the hCG.

Here is what I used of my own formulas:

Morning Regimen:

1) I used my formula called **Aloe Deep Cleanser.** *This is a botanical, organic base with oils, but they do not interfere or compromise the hCG protocol.* **It is completely water soluble**. *It goes on, is massaged a few minutes, and then comes off immediately with warm water and a cloth. When removed properly it* **leaves absolutely no oily residue** *and the skin is*

*squeaky clean. How do I know it is safe to use while doing the hCG system? I never had any weight gain by using my cleanser both **day and night**.*

Many don't realize that you should cleanse your face both night and morning. Your skin excretes or flushes the cells of excessive debris every eight hours. Therefore it very important you cleanse your face and neck every morning and night to help keep it radiant.

2) **Daily** I applied my **Isometric Face Lift with Aloe Activator**. *This is a totally unique program and can help normalize skin that is naturally either too dry or too oily. I have used this product virtually every morning since the mid-1970. Whereas I previously had extremely dry skin from living in the desert country years before, it is now smooth, clear, radiant, and virtually wrinkle free.*

*These products and application are so unique . . . it's a real example of: 'seeing is believing'. To demonstrate, I mix the isometric Lift Powder and Aloe Activator together, and then apply the lift mixture only on one side of their face. When it is removed 15 to 30 minutes later, the side that I **did not apply** the lift on,* *the person appears to have had a stroke on that side. The side where the lift was applied, all the fine wrinkles are either greatly diminished or have completely disappeared; deep creases are lessened; pores have shrunk measurably; the muscles and skin have visibly lifted; the skin is brighter, clearer and refreshed.* **The Lift program is oil free.**

3) Next I use my **Infinite Beauty Fluids.** *A totally oil-free mixture of active aloe vera, floral and herbal extracts, AHA and BHA that helps to renew and brighten your skin.*

4) Next I apply my **95% Aloe Hydrating Gel**. This is an oil-free gel that hydrates your skin without oils. *Only during the hCG protocol to I not use my regular* **Aloe Moisturizer** *or* **Night Nurture Creams** *due to their composition.*

5) I immediately applied my **Aloe OilFree Foundation while my skin was still slightly damp from the gel**. *This foundation is a soft creamy texture that protects your skin from the sun and environmental debris. We have an interesting test we can teach you can proving to yourself that my foundation is truly*

oilfree; or if you have another brand that claims to be 'oil free' you can verify if it is or not.

6) Next I apply my cheek and eye color along with my lipstick. I'm then set for whatever the day or evening requires. Seldom do I ever need to retouch my makeup, with the exception of my lipstick.

Evening Regimen:

I follow the same basic routine, but using only steps 1 – 3 – and 4 on the previous pages. If I feel like I need any type of extra moisture on my face, neck and hands I used a **tiny bit** of organic, cold-pressed virgin coconut oil. I only had to use it a couple of times due to exposure of extremely cold and dry weather. Coconut oil consists of median chain triglycerides *(MCT)* instead of the long chain triglycerides *(LCT)* as most other oils contain. The small amount of Coconut oil will not interfere with your hCG protocol **or** burning off your fat.

Coconut oil will generally be solid like a stick of butter. For convenience I put some in a small glass jar, and then set the jar in a cup of hot water when I needed to use it. It melts into actual oil at about 72-75° Fahrenheit or 22.2 – 23.88° Celsius.

If your skin gets too dry and flaky from showering or bathing, I suggest the following:

• Pore some organic apple cider vinegar in a squeeze bottle filling it only half full, and then finish filling the bottle with distilled water. Keep in the shower area. After you've showered and rinsed the soap off, squeeze a little of the vinegar around your shoulders from back to front, then rinse off. This will **remove** the soap residue which can cause irritation to your skin along with extreme dryness. *(FYI . . . this mixture helps re-establish the normal pH on your skin, which is slightly acid).*

• Use the **95% Aloe Gel** all over the body to sooth and hydrate. It will feel a little sticky for a moment until it absorbs into the skin. Let it air dry.

• If those two items mentioned previously aren't adequate to relieve your dry, itchy skin, then apply a little coconut oil. Be warned that a little goes a long way, so do not over use it.

Note: *Every time coconut oil is mentioned in this book I am referring only to Organic Cold-pressed Virgin Coconut Oil.* **Do not use hydrogenated coconut oil.**

As stated, most all other oils have LTC's and seem to stay in the body increasing your fat. Coconut Oil MTC's do not stay in the system but a very short time *(approximately 3 hours)* and do not cause the same damage as fats known as LTC's. *(For more information about Coconut Oil, you can request copies of my* **Innovations in Wellness** *Newsletter, the Jan and Feb, 2010 issues by emailing me at:* **Luci@InnovationsInWellness.com**).

Daily Grooming

While you are reducing may I suggest that you always groom yourself daily? You will be surprised how different it will make you feel. That is why I feel that using cosmetics is important. It helps build excitement within you each day as you weigh and groom yourself. You'll also get a lot more compliments, which makes you feel better about yourself, thus helping you keep going towards your ultimate goal. Weighing and grooming yourself should become a lifelong habit which should keep you on tract. See yourself as the beautiful or handsome person you are . . . and your reduction time will go much faster.

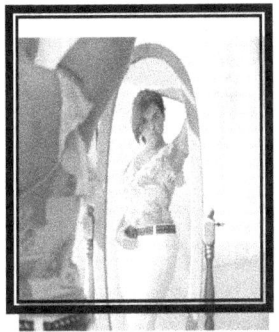 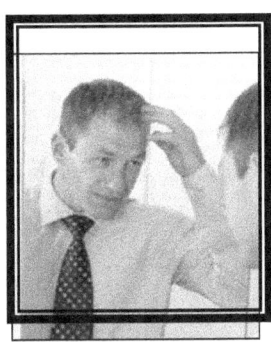

YOU ARE LOOKING GOOD . . .
GROOM EVERY DAY.

Conclusion– Congratulations

Did You Reach Your Goal?

I hope you have enjoyed and learned a lot about weight reduction and maintenance of your new slim and shapely body. By slim and shapely I'm talking about **curves for the women** and **muscles for the men** with reduction everywhere, especially the tummy.

The vital knowledge you've gained about your hypothalamus and its role in your overall wellbeing

should be of benefit to you for the rest of your life.

Sometimes it was hard to believe that for all those years I carried around the fat I hated. It's hard to believe that such **simple things** *as the* **hCG** *and the* **500 calorie diet** *could make so much difference so fast and so complete.*

Never before regardless of the exercise, diets, drinks, and pills, could I rid myself of that tummy fat, my thunder thighs, or my buttock.

I can now happily report that all that **fat is gone burned up and I intend to keep it that way.**

I owe so much thanks to Dr. Simeons and his miraculous discovery of hCG and subsequent 500 calorie diet.

My sincere appreciation and thanks to all of you who have purchased this book. I would love to hear from you and welcome any news of your successes. *Email your stories to:* **Luci@DontLoseFat-BurnIt.com**

Success comes to those who hope with a sincere desire, activate their faith and determination, and *then move forward to their ultimate goal knowing the beginning to the end.* ~Luci Flint

Free Offer ~ to all who ordered:

Don't Lose Fat ~ Burn It

If you would like to have more information on surprisingly healthy foods, oils, supplements and a few recipes that I use and endorse, I will gladly send it to you via **an e-zine** that is a complete booklet with the information that you can print off. All you need to do is send me an email requesting your free booklet:

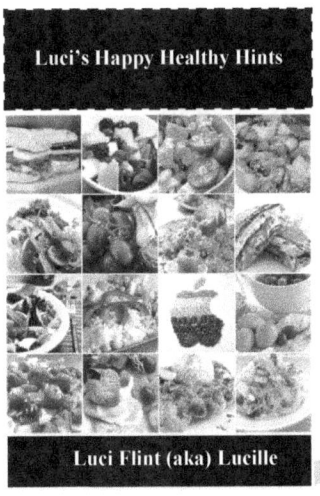

Email to: **Luci@HappyHealthyHints.com.**

(FYI . . . Purchase verification: I get a list of all purchasers

who bought the book along with their address and email, however you must include your address and email with your request).

I know this book will be given or loaned out to family or friends. Please don't, as you will need it to refer to often. Instead of giving them the ezine, suggest they acquire their own copy either by buying the book **'Don't Lose Fat ~ Burn It!** and ordering it free or by ordering their personal copy of:

Luci's Happy Healthy Hints

The cost is $10.00. Order it by sending a check or money order to:

Flint & Flint, LLC

P. O Box 496

New Harmony, UT 84757-0496.

P.S. Personal checks will have to clear the bank before the booklet is sent ~ please allow approximately two weeks. It's probably cheaper for them to order the book and get the ezine free.

I believe you all would also enjoy my **FREE** monthly newsletter **"Innovation In Wellness"**, which is chock full of: Fun Facts and Do You Know; Recipes; Questions and Answers; Articles about Health; New Products; New Ideas To Improve Yourself, etc.

If you would like to receive the newsletter or if you have any questions you would like to submit and have answered please send them via email to:

Luci@InnovationInWellness.com

If you have any favorite recipes you would like to share with others, please send them to the above email. *(You will receive acknowledgment for you contribution).*

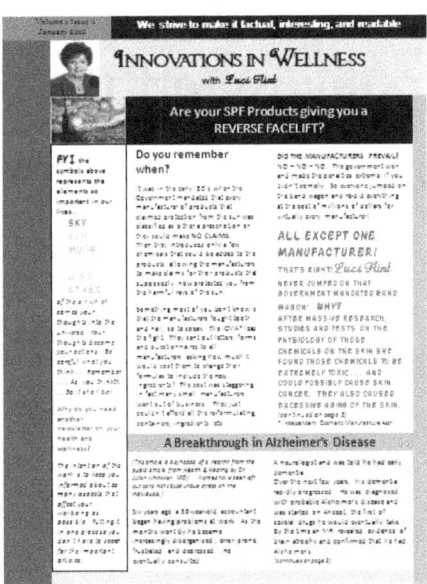

Twenty years from now you will be more disappointed by the things that you did not do than by the ones you did. So throw off the bowlines. Sail away from the safe harbor. Catch the trade winds in your sails to Discover ~ Explore ~ Dream

~ *Mark Twain*

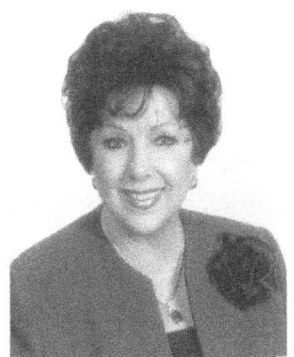

About the Author

Luci *(aka)* Lucille Flint is a highly trained and accomplished entrepreneur who is a successful leader, business strategist and organizational developer. She has visualized, implemented and started numerous successful businesses. Many of her ventures involve innovations into the well-being of others.

With over 50 years of real-world experience and extensive education; her down-to-earth connections are what make her the perfect choice to help you in your quest for a wellness, healthy life style, including **'reduction of weight by burning fat'**.

She has volunteered much of her resources and time to helping others in numerous and varied endeavors in their life, including many in foreign countries. The following is only a very brief summary of the plethora of accomplishments Lucille has achieved.

Lucille has been into the botanical, natural and organic movement since the late 1950's having studied, used and participated in virtually every health and wellness modality in that broad field.

Among numerous associations where she volunteered her time, Lucille served for nine years *(1979 -1989)* as an elected member of the National Executive Board for the National Nutritional Foods Association *(NNFA)*. The NNFA coordinates the 'Marketplace' every year uniting 'natural product' manufacturers, retailers and suppliers under one roof. Now uniting over 500 exhibitors lined up to inform and introduce their wares to each other and other registered contemporaries within the health and nutritional movement, especially the establishments known as 'Health Food Stores'.

In the 70's and 80's Lucille was part of the team that lobbied in Washington, D.C. to prevent the government from mandating that all vitamins, herbs and other supplements **be prescribed by doctors**.

With attorney, Milt Bass of New York City, they won their case and thanks to their heroic efforts you currently still have **freedom of choice** to determine what you want to take or not take, at least for now.

The following was written by a friend and associate, Betty Schenkey now deceased for Lucille 1985

She walks in beauty ~ She walks in light
She speaks truth ~ She speaks for you

She helps the downtrodden ~

She helps her friends

She loves unabashedly ~

She loves with no strings

She sees the good ~ She sees the light~
She prays for all ~ She prays for right
She is one with you ~ She is who she is~
She is our Lucille!

Be On The Alert ~

The government along with the AMA *(American Medical Association)* and drug companies are raising their greedy heads again. They want to again try to have legislation passed where you must have a **prescription to purchase any nutritional supplements**, including herbs, special health juices, etc. I feel that they want to control each phase of our lives as if we didn't have enough sense to take care of ourselves.

Get out there and fight for your rights to keep your 'Freedom of Choice'. Stop the FEDS who want to control every aspect of your life.

Freedom has its life in the hearts, the actions, the spirit of men and so it must be daily earned and refreshed – else like a flower cut from its life-giving roots, it will wither and die.

DISCLAIMER:

Whenever considering a weight loss program, consult with your physician or healthcare provider.

The information provided here is not intended to replace consultation or advice received from your doctor or qualified health professionals regarding your specific situation nor is it to be taken as medical advice or diagnosis. All information offered in this book are merely opinions regarding the diet proposed by Dr. Simeons. Losing 1 to 2 pounds a day is a result that many on the hCG diet have accomplished, but there is **NO GUARANTEE.** Nothing in this book should be considered as personalized health care advice.

Luci *(aka)* Lucille Flint, and/or any of her affiliates, associates or independent contractors shall NOT assume any legal, monetary, or any other type of responsibility for your decision to use this book as a guideline in the use of hCG and the 500 calorie diet or for any other reason.

*Luci does not receive any compensation for her recommendation of products, books and such that she has mentioned, **with exception** of the distribution of the **Lucille Flint Formulas** of which she receives a* *royalty.*

A smile is a language even
A baby understands.

It costs nothing
But it creates much.

It happens in a flash but the
Memory of it may last forever.

Keep on smiling!

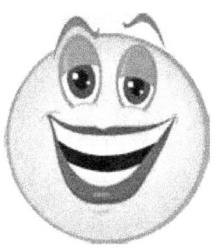

Bibliography

1) Weight Chart

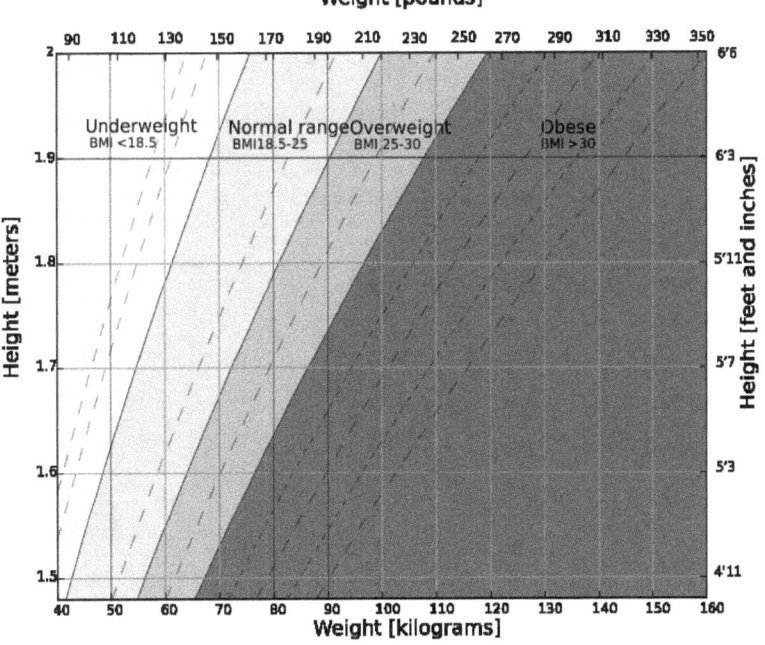

2) The information about hCG and 500 calories diet came from an article and papers written by Dr. A. T.W. Simeons,

"Pounds and Inches, A New Approach to Obesity"

3) Most of the information in the book is from research, studies, seminars, trainings, meetings, and practical experience by the author. Other information included in this book were taken from public information found while researching the subject, mostly on the internet, my own journals and books, which are too numerous to list.

4) Information concerning the hypothalamus was found in various articles found on the internet *(Wikipedia)*, and from my own medical books.

5) Pictures or photos were taken from Free Clip Art, with the exception of the cover, which was purchased.

6) Here are a few pictures for age comparisons *(un-retouched)*.

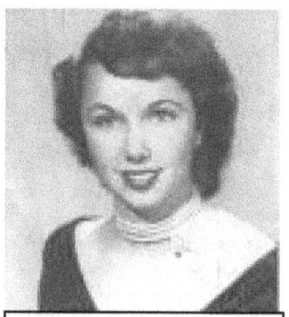

Age 19

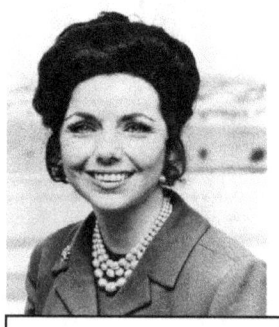

Age 35

Age 44 Passport
Photo

Age 54 Passport
Photo

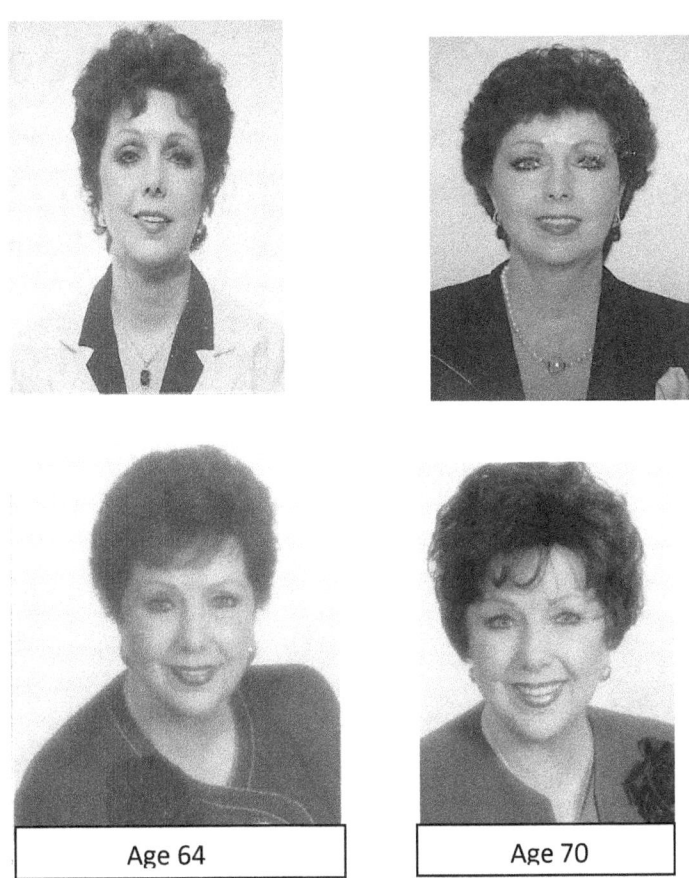

Age 64   Age 70

P.S. The photo at age 70 was taken in twenty minutes at a kiddie photo shop for a quick publicity shot. It was not retouched. This demonstrate the miraculous benefits her exclusive formulas.

The patriot's blood is

the seed of

Freedom's Tree.

~Thomas Campbell